# THE MINDSET DIET

# THE MINDSET DIET

Reframe your thinking and
transform your body for good

## GEORGIA HEINS

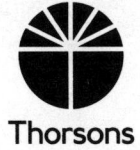

Thorsons

The information provided in this book is for educational and informational purposes only and is not intended as a substitute for professional medical advice, diagnosis, or treatment. Always seek the advice of your doctor or other qualified healthcare provider if you have any questions regarding a medical condition or treatment you know you have or suspect you may have. All efforts have been made to assure the accuracy of the information contained in this book as of the date of publication. However, please note that medical information can change over time and you should always seek to verify current medical standards.

Never disregard professional medical advice or delay in seeking it because of something you have read in this book. The author and publisher are not responsible for any adverse effects or consequences resulting from the use of any suggestions, preparations, or procedures discussed in this book and disclaim all liability in relation to the same. Reliance on any information provided in this book is solely at your own risk. If you think you are having a medical emergency, call the emergency services immediately.

Thorsons
An imprint of HarperCollins*Publishers*
1 London Bridge Street
London SE1 9GF

www.harpercollins.co.uk

HarperCollins*Publishers*
Macken House, 39/40 Mayor Street Upper
Dublin 1, D01 C9W8, Ireland

First published by Thorsons 2026

1 3 5 7 9 10 8 6 4 2

© Georgia Heins 2026

Georgia Heins asserts the moral right to be identified as the author of this work

A catalogue record of this book is available from the British Library

ISBN 978-0-00-878593-2

Printed and bound in the UK using 100% renewable electricity at CPI Group (UK) Ltd

All rights reserved. No part of this publication may be reproduced, stored in a retrieval system, or transmitted, in any form or by any means, electronic, mechanical, photocopying, recording or otherwise, without the prior written permission of the publishers.

Without limiting the exclusive rights of any author, contributor or the publisher of this publication, any unauthorised use of this publication to train generative artificial intelligence (AI) technologies is expressly prohibited. HarperCollins also exercise their |rights under Article 4(3) of the Digital Single Market Directive 2019/790 and expressly reserve this publication from the text and data mining exception.

# CONTENTS

Introduction: Flip the switch ..... 1

Chapter 1: Up Your Hydration Game ..... 14
Chapter 2: The Blood Sugar Sequence ..... 34
Chapter 3: Reclaiming the Night – the Value of Sleep ..... 56

Milestone 1 ..... 76

Chapter 4: The Balance Bank ..... 82
Chapter 5: The Hand-Portion Method ..... 98
Chapter 6: Shopping, Batching and 10-Minute Plates ..... 116
Chapter 7: Fun Foods Without the Negative Spiral ..... 136
Chapter 8: The Strength Code ..... 153
Chapter 9: The Training Mindset Shift ..... 175
Chapter 10: Cardio To Support Fat Loss – and Your Sanity ..... 194
Chapter 11: Your Psychological First-Aid Kit for Challenging Days ..... 210

Milestone 2 ..... 226

Chapter 12: Travel, Parties and Real Life ..... 230
Chapter 13: Back on Track in 24 Hours ..... 254
Chapter 14: The Identity Shift: Becoming You ..... 272

Milestone 3 ..... 287

Chapter 15: The Only Mindset You Need ..... 292

Afterword ..... 297

Reference Section ..... 301
Acknowledgements ..... 313
Notes ..... 314

# INTRODUCTION
# FLIP THE SWITCH

You know the moment. It's nine o'clock at night, the day has finally ended, the house is quiet, and a switch flips in your brain. You've been so 'good' all day. You had the sensible breakfast, you choked down the sad desk salad for lunch, you resisted the 3 p.m. sugar temptations. You've followed the rules. You've ticked the boxes. And now, standing in the soft, hopeful glow of the fridge light, a feeling of sheer exhaustion washes over you.

But it's not just tiredness. It's a deep, extreme fatigue from the constant effort of it all. The mental gymnastics, the willpower, the endless negotiations with yourself. And that's when the other voice kicks in. The one that's been quiet all day. 'Just one,' it whispers. 'Just one little square of chocolate. You've earned it.' Before you know it, the packet is empty, a familiar hot wave of guilt washing over you, and you're promising yourself that tomorrow you'll do better. You'll have more control. You'll be perfect.

For years, you've been trapped in this cycle. Starting over on Monday, feeling hopeful and motivated, only to find yourself derailed by Wednesday, defeated by Friday and promising to begin again next week. It's like your body AND your brain have teamed up against you – one craving chocolate, while your brain tells you you're a failure for wanting it. You've tried everything. You've counted the calories, tracked the points and eaten the 'clean' food. You've been to the classes, bought the workout plans and logged the 10,000 steps. And yet, you are still stuck. You are still battling the stubborn weight that clings around your middle, the energy crashes that sabotage your afternoons, the intense cravings that feel like an addiction, and the creeping feeling that your body is somehow broken. You look in the mirror and you don't see the vibrant, energetic woman you know you are on the inside. You feel disconnected, frustrated and unheard – especially by the doctors who tell you to just 'eat less and move more' – a common piece of advice which feels more like an insult.

So, you blame yourself. You decide you lack willpower. You believe you're not disciplined enough. You think you are the problem.

Let me be absolutely clear. Take a deep breath and let these words land:

*You* are not the problem.

The *rule book* is the problem.

You have been religiously following a set of rules that were never designed for your body. You have been fighting a battle against your own hormones, a battle you are biologically destined to lose.

And it is time to stop fighting. It is time to flip the switch.

This book is your new rule book. It is a fresh way of seeing and working with your body. In the following chapters I am going to share a simple, science-backed system that will enable you to finally stop the exhausting yo-yo cycle of dieting and get the results you've been working so hard for.

This is the last diet book you will ever need, because it is not a diet book. It is a user manual for your body.

I will show you how to work *with* your hormones, not against them; to unlock your energy and the body you've been fighting for; and give you the tools to maintain your results for life.

And I can make this promise with such certainty for one reason: I have lived every single moment of your frustration. This system didn't come from a textbook; it came from my own rock bottom.

## MY STORY: THE DIAGNOSIS THAT EXPLAINED EVERYTHING AND CHANGED NOTHING

On the outside, for most of my twenties, I looked healthy. I had what doctors call 'lean PCOS' (polycystic ovary syndrome). I was in a healthy weight range, I ate well, I exercised. But on the inside, I was at war with an invisible enemy.

The first sign was the puffiness: a constant, low-grade bloat that made my face round and my clothes feel tight. Then came the energy crashes. I'd wake up feeling tired after eight hours of sleep, force myself through the day with endless caffeine, and then collapse into a black hole of fatigue every afternoon around 3 p.m. Then there was my skin. My confidence was destroyed, one painful spot at a time, by cystic acne that spread across my chin and jawline. It was the kind of deep, sore acne that you can't cover with make-up, the kind that makes you want to cancel plans and hide your face from the world.

My rock bottom wasn't a number on the scale; it was a period of about three months when my skin was so bad, and my self-esteem so shattered, that I effectively became a hermit. I stopped going out with my friends, I made excuses to avoid social events and I cried myself to sleep most nights, my face throbbing, wondering what was wrong with me.

I remember one afternoon a delivery driver knocked on the door. My heart started pounding, I grabbed a baseball cap to pull down over my face and turned off all the lights in the hallway so he wouldn't be able to see me clearly when I opened the door.

That was the moment. Standing in the dark, hiding from the delivery driver, I realised I was living like a prisoner in my own life.

Getting diagnosed with polycystic ovary syndrome felt like a strange mix of relief and panic. Finally, these symptoms had a name. I wasn't going mental. The bloating, the spots, feeling absolutely knackered all the time, periods that showed up whenever they fancied – everything was connected. But that relief was overshadowed quickly by the bleak outlook described by the doctor.

He told me PCOS is a lifelong condition with no cure. He told me to lose some weight – advice that felt both insulting and impossible, given I was already a healthy size. He offered me hormonal medication, but scant explanation. I left his office with a crumpled leaflet and a feeling of dread so heavy it felt like a physical weight. I had a diagnosis, but I had no hope.

That night, I didn't cry. I got angry. And then I got curious. I opened my laptop and fell down a rabbit hole of medical journals, forums and scientific studies. And I was lucky. Through my social media platform, I was able to connect with leading doctors and researchers who thought differently to my doctor. And, slowly, through countless hours of research, I started to see a pattern. A word that kept appearing, a breadcrumb I followed, which led me to my 'Aha!' moment:

Insulin resistance.

I learned that most women with PCOS don't actually have a reproductive issue; they have a metabolic one. Research shows that three out of four women with PCOS have insulin resistance, which means their bodies are struggling to manage blood sugar.[1] This hormonal chaos is what creates all the downstream symptoms. My problem wasn't my ovaries; it was my blood sugar.

## INTRODUCTION

This was the lightbulb moment. My body wasn't broken. The insulin resistance was just sending it the wrong messages – constant blood sugar chaos that was throwing all my hormones out of whack. And if I could change those messages through what I ate and how I lived, maybe I could change everything.

But here's what's crucial – you don't need PCOS to struggle with insulin resistance. Research shows that insulin resistance affects millions of women, whether they have PCOS, are going through perimenopause, are chronically stressed or have affected their metabolism through years of restrictive dieting. The same insulin resistance that makes my PCOS body store fat when I eat irregularly affects millions of women, who will probably have been told their problem is 'lack of willpower'.

One of my clients, Tara, had been restricting her eating for so long that years of 1,200-calorie diets had made her metabolism adjust, which meant she now burned fewer calories, whatever she did. When she finally started eating enough her energy came back, the 3 p.m. crashes stopped and her body started responding normally again.

Jenny was 45 and thought perimenopause was her enemy. Her hormones were all over the place, her energy was crashing by midday and every diet made things worse. Turns out, her fluctuating oestrogen was creating insulin resistance – just like mine with PCOS. Once we started working with her hormone patterns instead of fighting them, everything clicked into place.

And Sarah? Stressed working mum, cortisol through the roof. That chronic stress was creating the exact same insulin resistance I have with PCOS. Her body was constantly in fight or flight mode, storing every carb as fat. Teaching her how to eat to manage cortisol changed everything – not just her weight, but her entire relationship with stress.

The point is this: whether it's PCOS, perimenopause, chronic stress or years of diet damage, the biology is the same. Your body stops listening to insulin properly. Food gets stored as fat instead of being used for energy. And you get told it's your fault for lacking willpower. It's not willpower. It's biology. And once you understand your specific biology, everything becomes possible.

This was the beginning of the system I'm going to share with you. A system that didn't just give me my body back; it gave me my life back.

## FIVE SIGNS YOUR BODY IS IN SURVIVAL MODE

Your body's number-one job is not to help you look good in a bikini, it's to keep you alive. When your body feels threatened – from stress, lack of sleep, unhealthy food – it switches to survival mode. And this means one thing for our bodies: storing fat like the apocalypse is coming.

Many of the symptoms you may be experiencing don't mean that you are failing. They are signs that your body feels unsafe:

1. **You have stubborn belly fat:** When your body is constantly stressed – from work, life or too much exercise and not enough food – it pumps out the stress hormone, cortisol, like it's going out of fashion. Your body's alarm bell is screaming 'CRISIS!', signalling to your body to store emergency fuel. So that stubborn little pouch around your middle isn't there because you're lazy, it's your body banking fat to try to keep you alive.
2. **You have intense cravings:** When your blood sugar crashes after a poor meal, your brain goes into panic mode and demands the fastest fuel it can get – sugar. But this creates more blood sugar chaos, not stability. This is your body's SOS signal. But you're not broken, your body is just under stress.

3. **You eat 'perfectly' and get no results:** This is the ultimate sign. If you are undereating and exercising hard and the dial is not moving, your body is sending you a clear message. It has adapted to your low intake by slowing down your metabolism to conserve energy because it thinks you aren't getting enough food.
4. **You obsess about food constantly:** When your body feels deprived, it increases mental absorption with food as a survival mechanism. That constant thinking about your next meal, planning what you'll eat or feeling guilty about food choices isn't lack of willpower – it's your brain trying to ensure you don't 'starve'. Your body is keeping food front and centre in your thoughts to protect you from what it perceives as famine.
5. **You are chronically fatigued:** Look, everyone gets a bit of an energy dip around 3 p.m. – that's just our natural body clock. But the dramatic crashes many women experience? That's something else entirely. Constant exhaustion, especially that 'I need sugar ASAP' feeling, is a classic symptom of a body struggling with its energy system. You're living on a blood sugar rollercoaster instead of having steady, balanced fuel.

Your body is not fighting you. It is trying to protect you. Our job is not to punish it further; our job is to finally make it feel safe. Your old habits have led you to this place. The yo-yo dieting, the work stress, the sleepless nights, the missed gym sessions, the dehydration, the misinformation. Your body's default setting is in survival mode. Let's change that together, right now.

## THE HIDDEN GUT–STRESS CONNECTION

Your gut health and stress response are more connected than you might think. When you're chronically stressed – from work pressures, family demands or constantly fighting your body with restrictive dieting – your digestive system takes a massive hit.

Here's what happens: stress hormones like cortisol literally change your gut bacteria. The 'good' bacteria that help regulate your appetite, mood and inflammation get wiped out, while the 'bad' bacteria that promote cravings and weight gain take over. And this isn't just about bloating or digestive issues (though those are real, too). Your gut produces 90 per cent of your body's serotonin – the 'happy hormone' that also regulates sleep and appetite. When your gut is stressed and inflamed, your entire hormone system goes haywire.

Tara noticed this connection immediately. Years of restrictive dieting had left her with constant digestive issues, brain fog and those evening cravings she couldn't control. When we worked on healing her gut alongside supporting her metabolism, not only did her digestion improve, her energy came back, her sleep improved and those 3 p.m. sugar crashes disappeared entirely.

Your gut isn't separate from your weight struggles – it's central to them.

## WHY EVERYTHING HURTS (INFLAMMATION)

If you feel like your body is constantly fighting against you – achy joints, puffy face, swollen fingers, stubborn weight that won't budge – you're likely dealing with chronic inflammation.

This isn't the helpful inflammation that heals a cut or fights off an infection. This is your body's alarm system stuck in the 'on' position, creating a constant state of internal fire.

What triggers this chronic inflammation?

- Chronic stress. (Hello, constant dieting and self-criticism …)
- Ultra-processed foods that your body sees as foreign invaders.

- Poor sleep from stress and blood sugar crashes.
- Over-exercising while under-eating (yes, this is inflammatory).
- Gut health issues that leak inflammatory molecules into your bloodstream.

When your body is inflamed, weight loss becomes nearly impossible. Inflammation promotes fat storage, disrupts hormone signals and makes your body hold on to water like it's preparing for drought.

Laura (see page 15) always said she felt like a 'pufferfish'. Despite eating perfectly and exercising religiously, she felt swollen and uncomfortable in her own skin. Once we addressed the inflammation through stress management, gut healing and proper nutrition timing, she lost two dress sizes in eight weeks – not through restriction, but through healing.

Your body isn't broken or lazy. It's inflamed and trying to protect you.

## WHAT IS YOUR DRIVING FORCE?

Before we talk about any of the practical strategies in this book, I need to ask you something crucial: what are your core values?

Or, to put that another way, what's your North Star?

I don't mean your weight-loss goal or your target dress size. I mean the deeper reason why you picked up this book. The real why behind the why.

Maybe you're embarking on this journey so you can chase your toddler around the playground without getting winded. Maybe it's so you feel confident and radiant in photos at your daughter's wedding. Maybe it's so you can model genuine self-care for the people you love, showing them what it looks like to treat your body as a trusted partner rather than an enemy.

Ideally, your North Star shouldn't be about fitting into jeans from ten years ago. Ideally, it would be about who you want to become and how you want to feel as you move through your life.

## THE PROBLEM WITH GOALS (AND WHY THEY EXPIRE)

For years, your 'why' was probably a goal. An outcome. Something like:

- 'I want to lose a stone for my holiday.'
- 'I want to fit into my old jeans.'
- 'I want to look good for that wedding.'

Goals are great for getting you started, but they have one fatal flaw: an expiry date. A holiday is a week. A wedding is a day. The second the event is over, your 'why' vanishes. And without a 'why,' the motivation dies, and the habits crumble.

Your North Star is different, it is your value code. It's not a destination you arrive at. It's a direction you travel in, forever.

## WHAT'S YOUR NORTH STAR?

Take a moment. Look at these words: health, freedom, strength, presence. Maybe your North Star is one of them. Maybe it's another word entirely, like 'confidence', 'vitality' or 'peace'. What is the one value that you are truly wedded to? What is the 'why' that will get you out of bed on a cold morning and guide you through a tough choice?

Write it down. This is your North Star. When your motivation fades – and it will – you will no longer ask, 'Do I feel like it?' You will ask, 'Does this action move me closer to my North Star?' That is a question with a much clearer answer. And it's a source of fuel that will never, ever run out.

## WHY IS IT SO IMPORTANT?

Your North Star – your core value – shapes the identity you choose to embody. That identity then drives the daily behaviours that become your life. When these three elements align, change becomes effortless because you're not fighting against yourself anymore.

For example: if your North Star is 'Being a strong role model for my children,' you might choose the identity of 'The woman who takes care of herself.' That identity then naturally leads to behaviours like choosing nourishing meals and moving your body regularly – not because you have to, but because that's simply what that woman chooses to do, and does.

The strategies in this book – the mindset shifts, the meal frameworks, the movement principles – they're all just vehicles to get you there. They're tools in service of something much bigger than weight loss. They're pathways to your North Star.

So, let's start exploring those pathways.

## THE SECRET IS IN SIMPLICITY

This book is built around four simple, powerful 'metabolic switches'. These are not complicated rules. They are small, strategic shifts in *how* and *when* you do things. They are designed to send a new set of signals to your body – to make it feel safe. When you start flipping these switches, you move your body out of survival mode and into a state of high energy, and effortless fat-burning.

Here are the changes we will make:

1. **The water-timing secret:** You've been told to drink more water. But no one had told you that *when* you drink it is crucial. This tiny shift boosts your energy, eases sugar cravings and puts an

end to that uncomfortable bloating from water retention that makes your jeans feel tight.
2. **The craving-control code:** A simple food-order formula that balances your blood sugar and stops cravings before they even begin. This isn't about restriction; it's about strategic, science-backed timing.
3. **The 3-day burn:** What if working out *less* (yep, just three times a week) could speed up fat loss more? This flips everything you thought you knew about daily workouts and builds a lean, strong body on your terms, without the burnout.
4. **The overnight fat-loss switch:** A one-tweak evening routine that resets your appetite, calms your hormones and turns your sleep into a secret fat-burning weapon.

What can you expect? In the first seven days of applying these principles, you will not be 'perfect', and you will not lose 10 pounds. This is not a quick fix. But you will notice you have more energy. You will notice your cravings are quieter. You will notice you feel less bloated and puffy. You will get a glimpse of what it feels like to have a body that is working *with* you. And that feeling is the most powerful motivation on the planet.

## HOW TO SUCCEED THIS TIME: THE 2-MINUTE GOAL

Most approaches fail because they expect you to become a completely different person overnight. They expect you to completely overhaul your relationship with food, exercise and your body in one giant leap. Instead, we're going to start small. So small you'll feel a bit silly, but so small it's very easily achievable.

Our guiding principle will be the idea of small, achievable goals. Proven to work and easy to remember: any new habit must take less than two minutes to start.

Want to drink more water? → Start with one glass when you wake up.

Want to exercise more? → Put your trainers next to your bed to put on in the morning.

Want to eat a better diet? → Add one vegetable to your plate of food.

Why? Because at the start, we're not chasing results – we're chasing consistency. We're trying to prove to ourselves that we're the kind of person who follows through. We want to make good habits stick. Every tiny action is like a vote for who you're becoming. Two minutes of meditation? That's you voting to be someone who cares about their mental health. One sentence in a journal? That's you voting to be someone who reflects and grows.

We cannot fail if we stick to our achievable goals: those daily, small steps that build success and momentum. It's that momentum that'll carry you through, until conscious motivation isn't needed anymore, as it's simply evolved into good habits.

As a 'read-then-do' guide, this book is designed around the idea of small goals. At the end of each chapter, you will find a simple, clear action plan. Your job is to do that one thing. That is how you win.

# CHAPTER 1
# UP YOUR HYDRATION GAME

Let's talk about that water bottle. You know the one. It's massive – almost a small bucket, with motivational quotes slapped on the side. 'You've got this!' 'Keep chugging!' An embarrassment, but you carry it everywhere anyway. It's glued to your hand or sits on your desk, like a virtue-signalling trophy telling everyone you're being healthy. You sip away all day, tick your little hydration boxes, and feel satisfied when you drain the last drop. By all accounts, you're absolutely smashing this hydration thing.

So why do you feel so ... rubbish? Why do your fingers feel like sausages, making your rings so tight on your fingers that you have to clench and unclench your fists? Why do you feel so bloated from water retention that by the end of the day you have to undo the top button of your jeans on the drive home, your stomach feeling like a sloshing, uncomfortable water balloon? Why are you hit so hard by a wave of exhaustion mid-afternoon that you would consider selling a kidney for a 15-minute nap under your desk? Why do your sugar cravings still feel like a primal, uncontrollable urge, a goblin in your brain screaming for biscuits? And why, for the love of God, are you peeing every forty-five minutes? You've been to the loo more times than you've answered emails, and your urine is running crystal clear. You even thought that was a good thing.

You're doing exactly what you've been told to do. You're drinking the water. So why isn't it *working*?

If this is you – if you've ever felt deeply frustrated about doing everything right but getting nowhere – then listen up. You're not going mad. The problem isn't that you're not drinking enough water. The problem is that you've only been told half the story. You've been told to fill the tank, but nobody has ever told you how to get the fuel into the engine. You've been trying to solve the wrong problem.

It's not about *how much* water you're drinking – it's about whether your body can *use* it.

And – spoiler alert – it can't. You've been concentrating on the volume of water, when in fact you need to rethink hydration and focus on absorption instead.

### LAURA'S STORY

This brings me to my client, Laura. A brilliant mum of three, the CEO of her family, she looked like she had it all sorted. Her kids' diaries were colour-coded masterpieces – swimming lessons, playdates, perfectly packed lunches. They always had matching socks. A spotless house, her life was planned to the minute, and always sitting on her kitchen counter was a huge two-litre water bottle that she'd religiously refill at least once a day. She was ticking all the boxes.

When she came to me, her main complaint was a constant, bone-deep tiredness that made no sense.

'I don't get it,' she said on our first call, her voice a mix of exhaustion and frustration I know so well from knackered mums. 'I get eight hours of sleep, I eat my salads, I drink four litres of water a day. I should have amazing energy, but I feel like I'm

> wading through treacle. And I'm so bloated, all the time. I feel like a human pufferfish. I have to unbutton my jeans by midday and hide the evidence under a baggy jumper, hoping no one notices. It's miserable.'
>
> I asked her to describe her hydration routine. 'Simple,' she said. 'I chug. I start with a pint of plain water as soon as I wake up and I don't stop until I go to bed.'
>
> I then asked, 'When you wake up, are you thirsty?'
>
> Laura looked at me, confused. 'Desperate,' she replied. 'My mouth is like the Sahara Desert. That's why I have the pint of water first thing.'

That was the clue. I explained to Laura that despite drinking four litres of water, she was, on a cellular level, profoundly dehydrated. By that, I mean the water wasn't getting *inside* the trillions of tiny cells that make up her muscles, her brain and her organs, which is where it needs to be to create energy. Instead, her 'chugging' was just creating that 'sloshing' in her system, leading to the puffiness and the constant trips to the loo. But it wasn't being *absorbed*. She was effectively drowning in water, while her cells were dying of thirst.

## THE SCIENCE PART: UNDERSTANDING HYDRATION

To understand why you feel like a human pufferfish despite your best hydration efforts, we need to know that there are two places where water can be in your body: *inside* your cells, and *outside* your cells.

- **The goal – cellular hydration:** This is where the magic happens. When water is inside your cells, it powers your mitochondria (your tiny cellular energy factories), facilitates nutrient transport,

and keeps your entire system running efficiently. This is what makes you feel energetic, clear-headed and vibrant. Your skin is plump, your brain is sharp and your energy level is stable.
- **The problem – extracellular hydration:** This is the water that is 'sloshing' around in the spaces *between* your cells. When you have too much water here and not enough inside your cells, you feel puffy, bloated and heavy. This is the water that makes your rings tight and your ankles swell.

This is not just about bloating. A lack of cellular hydration is directly connected to your two biggest frustrations: uncontrollable cravings and stalled fat loss.

## WHY DEHYDRATION FEELS LIKE A SUGAR CRAVING

Have you ever noticed how your most intense sugar cravings hit around 3 p.m., right when your brain starts feeling like mush? It's no coincidence. Here's what's happening: the hypothalamus is the part of your brain that controls both hunger and thirst. When you're dehydrated, the wires get crossed. Your brain knows it needs energy, fast, but instead of asking for water, it screams for sugar.

You don't have a willpower problem. You've got a communication problem. Your body's asking for water, but your brain's hearing 'emergency biscuits required'. So, when you rethink your hydration – getting water into your cells instead of just sloshing around them – you give your brain what it needs. And that craving goblin that's been yelling at you all afternoon? It finally goes quiet.

## WHY A DEHYDRATED BODY WON'T BURN FAT

Your body's got one job: to keep you alive. When it thinks you're dehydrated, it panics and goes into full survival mode.

Think about a houseplant you've forgotten to water – does it waste energy trying to grow lovely new leaves? Of course not. It goes into crisis mode, stops growing, wilts and clings to every drop of water it's got left. Your body reacts in the same way. When it's dehydrated at a cellular level, it assumes there's a crisis happening. Cortisol starts pumping, stress levels go through the roof and your body thinks, 'We're in survival mode now. No way am I burning fat when we might be running out of food.'

> ### CORTISOL: THE HORMONE EVERYONE IS TALKING ABOUT
>
> **What is cortisol anyway?** Cortisol is your body's built-in alarm system – think of it as your internal fire brigade. When there's a genuine emergency (like a tiger chasing you or, in the modern world, a work deadline), cortisol floods your system to get you moving. Heart rate up, blood sugar up, focus sharp – it's brilliant in actual survival situations.
>
> **Why is everyone losing their minds about it?** Because we're treating everyday life like a constant emergency. That work email at 9 p.m.? Cortisol spike. Instagram comparison scrolling? Cortisol spike. Skipping meals then binge eating? Massive cortisol spike. Your body can't tell the difference between a real threat and you stressing about your to-do list.
>
> **What happens when cortisol's constantly elevated?**
> - You store fat around your middle (because your body thinks you're about to starve).
> - Sleep is disrupted because you can't switch off.
> - Cravings for sugar and carbs go crazy (quick energy needed for the 'emergency').

- Your immune system takes a beating.
- Brain fog becomes your constant companion.

**The evening cortisol problem:** Cortisol should naturally drop in the evening as melatonin (your sleepy hormone) rises. But when you're scrolling your phone, working late, or having sugar before bed, you're telling your body: 'STAY ALERT! DANGER!' when it should be winding down.

**The fix isn't complicated:** Respect your cortisol rhythm instead of fighting it. Morning cortisol peak = good for energy and focus. Evening cortisol drop-off = essential for sleep and recovery. Work with it, not against it.

When your cells are properly hydrated, your body receives a different message: 'We're safe. We've got plenty. You can relax and let go of this stored energy.'

So, here's the key question: how do you get water into your cells instead of just swilling around outside them, making you feel like a waterlogged sponge?

The answer is minerals. Specifically, electrolytes.

## ANALOGY: THE WORLD'S MOST EXCLUSIVE HOUSE PARTY

Imagine your body is like a massive house party. There are trillions of little VIP rooms – your cells – where all the good stuff happens: the energy, the buzz, all of it. Now, all that water you're chugging religiously? That's like hundreds of people turning up to this party, all queuing in the hallway, desperate to get into the VIP rooms where the real party's happening.

But here's the problem. In the 'just drink more water' world, we keep shoving more people into that hallway. It gets crowded.

Everyone's squashed, can't move, having a rubbish time. That's your bloating – all that chaos in the hallway.

And when nobody can get into the VIP party rooms, they eventually become fed up and leave the house altogether. That's you peeing out all that water you've been dutifully drinking.

So, how do we get people out of the packed hallway and into the party rooms?

We need the hosts. They have got the keys to all the VIP rooms. Their job is to stand at the doors, open them up, personally inviting guests inside. Without the hosts, those doors stay locked tight, no matter how many people are crushed in the hallway.

In your body, these hosts are called electrolytes – minerals like sodium, potassium and magnesium. When you drink plain water, you're just adding more people to the hallway situation. But when you drink water with the right minerals, you're allowing the hosts to open the doors and escort the water to where it belongs – inside your cells, where it can get to work.

## MEET THE HOSTS: YOUR MINERAL A-TEAM

Salt has been the nutritional bad guy for decades. We've been told to fear it, to cut it out, that it's the cause of all our problems. And while it's true that the highly processed, bleached-white table salt found in junk food isn't your friend, the natural and unrefined salt from the sea or the mountains is not just a good guy, it is the hero of our story.

- **Sodium (the head doorman):** Sodium is the guy in charge. He controls what happens outside your cells – manages who gets into the hallway in the first place. Without enough sodium, your body thinks, 'No, we don't need this water,' and sends it straight back out. That's why you can drink litres of the stuff and still feel parched. You need the sodium to get the party started.

- **Potassium (the VIP room manager):** Potassium is sodium's partner in crime, but he works inside your cells. He's in the VIP rooms, opening doors from the inside, pulling people in from that crowded hallway. These two work together as a team – it's called the sodium-potassium pump, which sounds fancy, but it just means they maintain a balance between them.
- **Magnesium (the calm party planner):** If sodium and potassium are your door staff, magnesium is the event manager making sure everything runs smoothly. This mineral is involved in more than 300 different jobs in your body, including energy production and blood sugar control. Most importantly, it keeps your nervous system chilled out. The problem is that most of us are running on empty with magnesium. It's like when your party planner goes AWOL – suddenly everything feels chaotic and stressful.

In fact, current hydration advice tells us to do the two things that completely mess up our mineral A-Team, by telling us to 1. chug loads of plain, filtered water that contains zero minerals and washes out the ones we have already, and 2. avoid salt like it's going to kill us.

It's as if we've fired all our party staff and then wonder why the whole event is a disaster.

Our goal is to adopt a food-first philosophy, by getting these crucial minerals from our diet, not just from powders and pinches of salt.

## SODIUM: THE HEAD DOORMAN

**The why:** Most people think they need to avoid sodium, but that's only half true. We get plenty of processed sodium from packaged foods but we often lack the right kind of sodium that works with potassium. Quality sodium helps your body actually hold on to the water you drink instead of just flushing it straight through. You can find this unrefined sea salt or rock salt in most health shops and larger supermarkets – look for labels that say 'unrefined' or 'natural'.

## POTASSIUM: THE VIP ROOM MANAGER

**The why:** Potassium works closely with sodium, but it does its job inside our cells. Both need to work together harmoniously for your nerves to operate properly and for your muscles to do their thing. The challenge is that many of us are only getting processed sodium from junk food, and barely any potassium from real food, which messes up the balance between this duo.

**How to get it:** Focus on colourful, whole plant foods – your potassium powerhouses.

- **Avocado:** The undisputed king. Half an avocado packs a huge potassium punch.
- **Leafy greens:** Spinach and Swiss chard are excellent sources.
- **Potatoes and sweet potatoes:** Yes, potatoes! A baked potato (with the skin on) is loaded with potassium.
- **Coconut water:** A brilliant natural source, which helps stabilise blood sugar and reduce afternoon cravings.
- **Bananas and oranges:** Classic choices for a reason.

> ### MAGNESIUM: THE CALM PARTY PLANNER
>
> **The why:** Magnesium is the ultimate relaxation mineral. It helps to calm the nervous system, relax our muscles and is critical for blood sugar regulation. Stress depletes magnesium like a hole in a bucket, and most of us are running on empty.
>
> **How to get it:**
>
> - **Dark chocolate:** Good quality dark chocolate (70 per cent cocoa or higher) is a fantastic and delicious source.
> - **Nuts and seeds:** Almonds, cashews and pumpkin seeds are at the top of the list.
> - **Legumes:** Black beans and edamame are great options.
> - **Epsom salt baths:** Your skin is your biggest organ. Soaking in a bath with Epsom salts (magnesium sulphate) is a wonderful way to absorb magnesium and calm your system before bed.
>
> By consciously including these foods (or rituals) in your life, you are hosting a resilient, well-staffed cellular party, every single day.

## YOUR HYDRATION SYSTEM

Choose your electrolytes wisely, as not all salt is created equal. Select the good stuff: unrefined options like Celtic sea salt or Himalayan pink salt. They contain not just sodium but also a rich spectrum of trace minerals, including magnesium and potassium. This is the complete party-planning team.

Electrolyte powders can be fantastic but read the label like a detective. Look for brands that are primarily sodium, potassium and magnesium. Avoid powders that list 'sugar' or 'fructose' as the first ingredient. Many popular sports drinks are just sugary junk food disguised as a health product.

Here are four key steps to turn you from a water-chugger into a cellular hydrator.

## 1. THE MORNING SALT ELIXIR KICKSTART (THE MOST IMPORTANT STEP)

The first thing you put into your body in the morning sets the tone for the entire day. After seven to eight hours of sleeping, breathing and repairing, you wake up in a state of dehydration. That feeling of morning grogginess and the immediate craving for caffeine is your body screaming for water and minerals.

**What to do:** Before you do anything after waking up, you are going to drink a large glass of water (around 500ml) with a pinch of good-quality, unrefined sea salt or rock salt dissolved in it (see page 30).

This does two things. The water provides the guests, and the salt provides the head doorman (sodium) that tells your body, 'Hold on to this water; we need it. Let's get this party started.' It allows the water to be absorbed into your system, providing an immediate, noticeable boost in energy and mental clarity, often within minutes.

## 2. SUPPORT YOUR WORKOUT

When you exercise, you sweat. And sweat isn't just water; it's water and salt.

**What to do:** About 30 minutes before you exercise, have another glass of salted water. This pre-loads your system with the minerals it's about to lose, ensuring your muscles and nerves can fire efficiently.

## 3. THE MID-AFTERNOON 'MEH'

That 3 p.m. slump is almost always a mini-dehydration crisis. Your brain is low on energy, and it sends out the signal for the fastest possible fuel: sugar. Before you reach for a biscuit, address the root cause.

**What to do:** Create an afternoon elixir. In a glass of water, mix a pinch of sea salt and a squeeze of lemon or a splash of coconut water (a great source of potassium). This rehydrates you on a cellular level and can often stop an energy slump and a sugar craving in its tracks.

## 4. PREPARING FOR A GOOD NIGHT'S SLEEP

You can help yourself in the evening, too, by preparing your body for a good night's sleep and a good morning the following day.

**What to do:** About two hours before bed, have a small glass of water with a pinch of sea salt. This helps maintain cellular hydration overnight and supports the body's natural wind-down process. When your electrolyte balance is steady, your nervous system stays calm – and your sleep quality improves.

# ELECTROLYTE POWDERS VS. UNREFINED SALT: WHAT YOU'RE REALLY GETTING

| Feature | Celtic Sea Salt | Most Electrolyte Powders |
| --- | --- | --- |
| Ingredients | Single ingredient: unrefined salt packed with 80+ trace minerals | Multiple synthetic additives, sweeteners, 'natural' flavours, preservatives |
| Hormone impact | Hormone-neutral (supports adrenal and electrolyte balance) | Often includes fillers that spike insulin or disrupt gut-hormone signalling |
| Gut health | Supports digestion and stomach acid production | Can irritate the gut lining |
| Hydration effect | Pulls water into cells for deep, lasting hydration | May cause frequent urination without true cellular hydration |
| Taste | Neutral or lightly salty; easy to mask | Artificially sweet; often contains sucralose, or flavour-masking agents |
| Daily use safety | Safe for regular use in small amounts | Not ideal for daily use due to sweeteners and additives |
| Purpose | Everyday mineral support | Designed for high-performance athletes or medical rehydration |

# YOUR NO-NONSENSE FAQs

### 'But isn't salt bad for my blood pressure?'

This is an important question, and I need to be straight with you here. All that 'salt is evil' advice comes from studies of people eating poor diets with barely any potassium, and using processed table salt. The science is changing, though. Experts now believe that the balance between sodium and potassium is crucial, not just avoiding salt completely. The real problem with how most people eat is we're getting too much processed sodium from junk food, but not any potassium from vegetables and fruits.

Our protocol is different. Taking in proper, unrefined sea salt – with all the trace minerals still in it – alongside a diet including potassium from foods such as avocados and leafy greens will achieve the right balance. This is very different from a diet including lots of processed table salt.

That said, if you have been diagnosed with high blood pressure or any kidney condition, you should speak to your doctor before increasing your salt intake.

### 'I'm peeing every five minutes! How long does this take to work?'

Welcome to the adaptation phase! If you are a water-chugger, your body has become used to getting rid of water as fast as it comes in. It's trained itself to think, 'Oh, here we go again, more pointless water – out you go.'

When you start including minerals, your body needs time to catch up and realise what's happening. For most people, this 'living in the loo' phase only lasts about three to five days. Stick with it – I promise it's worth it.

Once your body trusts you to give it the minerals it needs, it'll start hanging on to water where it belongs. You'll go from peeing every hour to being able to sit through a meeting without planning your escape route to the toilets.

### 'What about sparkling water, diet drinks and juices?'

Sparkling water: great! It's just water with carbonation. It's just as hydrating as still water.

Diet drinks: These are a grey area. While they don't contain sugar, the intense artificial sweeteners can still mess with your gut microbiome and, for some people, trigger an insulin response and cravings. Think of them as a 'better than' option compared to a sugary drink, but not as good as water.

Fruit juice: Treat this as a sugar source, not a hydration source. When you remove the juice from the fruit, you remove all the fibre, leaving you with a concentrated hit of fructose that will spike your blood sugar. Eat whole fruit instead.

### 'I get headaches when I start this. What's going on?'

Headaches can happen when you're changing your electrolyte balance, especially if you've been avoiding salt for ages. It's usually just your body adjusting – annoying, but temporary.

Make sure you're not overdoing the salt. We're talking a pinch in 500ml water. Plus, double check you're getting your potassium and magnesium from food, not just focusing on the sodium.

If the headaches stick around or get worse, ease off and have a chat with a medical professional. Your body's always the boss. If it's telling you something's not right, listen to it.

### 'What about coffee and tea? Do they count?'

Yes, they are mostly water. The old myth that they are dehydrating is largely debunked. However, caffeine is a mild diuretic, so stick to the 'one for one' rule: for every cup of coffee or tea you drink, have a glass of mineralised water alongside.

> **FOR HORMONAL BALANCES**
>
> If you struggle with a hormonal imbalance – whether that's PCOS, perimenopause, or just feeling like your cycle's all over the place – getting your mineral balance sorted is even more important, as your body's ability to stabilise blood sugar and manage stress is directly linked to how well you're hydrated at a cellular level.

> **A helpful tweak:** Try waiting 60 to 90 minutes after waking before you have your first coffee. Have your morning salt water elixir first. This lets your natural morning cortisol settle before adding caffeine, which can lead to having calmer, more stable energy all day.

## A 24-HOUR HYDRATION TIMELINE

Let's walk through a full day, comparing the old hydration way with the new.

### *Waking up*
- **Old way:** Mouth like a desert. You feel groggy and irritable until your first coffee.
- **New way:** You have your morning salt water elixir. Within minutes, you feel a gentle, clear energy. The brain fog lifts.

### *Mid-morning*
- **Old way:** You're on your second coffee, feeling a bit jittery, and you've already been to the loo three times.
- **New way:** You feel calm and focused. You sip your mineralised water. Your energy is stable.

### *3 p.m. slump*
- **Old way:** You hit the wall. Your brain feels like sludge. The biscuit tin is calling your name.
- **New way:** You have your craving-crusher afternoon elixir. The fog lifts, the craving subsides and you power through your afternoon.

### Evening

- **Old way:** You feel puffy and bloated. Your rings are tight.
- **New way:** You feel light and your stomach is calm. You're winding down, not bloating up.

This isn't magic. It's just biology. It's the feeling of a body that is finally, truly hydrated from the inside out. We have cleared the fog and turned the power on at a cellular level.

I know some of you are probably reading this and pulling a face at the thought of drinking more water, let alone salty water. I get it. Plain water can be boring, but here's the thing ... you don't have to suffer, as there are loads of ways to get your minerals in without it tasting like you're gargling seawater.

For those who are sensitive to the taste of salt – start small. We're talking a tiny pinch that you can barely taste (you actually shouldn't be able to taste it). Your taste buds will adapt over a week or two, then you can gradually add a bit more.

> **NATURAL FLAVOUR BOOSTERS**
>
> These aren't just going to make your water taste nicer – they're adding extra minerals and benefits, too.
>
> - **Lemon or lime water** – squeeze half a lemon into your salt water. The vitamin C helps with mineral absorption and masks any salty taste.
> - **Ginger lemon** – grate fresh ginger into your water with lemon juice. Brilliant for digestion and the zingy taste will cover up any mineral flavour.

- **Cucumber mint water** – slice up a cucumber and throw in some fresh mint. Cucumber is loaded with potassium, and mint makes everything feel more refreshing.
- **Berry water** – add a handful of frozen berries to your bottle. As they defrost, they'll flavour the water and add antioxidants. Frozen will give a better taste than fresh.
- **Apple cinnamon** – slice an apple, add a cinnamon stick. Feels like you're drinking something fancy, plus cinnamon helps regulate your blood sugar.
- **Coconut water** – this is basically nature's sports drink. It's naturally high in potassium and has a sweet taste. Mix it half and half with regular water and add a pinch of salt for extra hydration – job done.

Correct hydration is our foundation. We have deep-dived into that most important metabolic switch: what to drink and when to drink it, to optimise how you feel. I've shown you why that feeling of being constantly puffy and bloated from water retention has nothing to do with what you're eating, and everything to do with when you are drinking.

We are going to make your body feel safe, hydrated and energised, from the inside out.

# YOUR FIRST ACTION PLAN: HYDRATE LIKE A PRO

**The mindset shift:** Every sip is supporting your body's natural processes – you're not maintaining a habit, you're maintaining yourself.

**The task:** Go to your kitchen cupboard. If you see fine, white, iodised table salt, get rid of it. Next time you are at the shops, your only mission is to buy a bag of unrefined sea salt or Himalayan pink salt. This is your new kitchen staple.

**The practice:** Every morning this week, start your day with the morning salt water elixir (500ml water + a pinch of good salt). If you struggle with hormones, also try the 90-minute caffeine delay every morning this week. For the rest of the day stick to plain water, as your morning dose has set you up perfectly.

**If exercising:** Add a pinch of your new salt to your main water bottle.

**The 3 p.m. check-in:** When the afternoon slump hits, have your afternoon elixir *before* you reach for a snack.

At the end of each day this week, track your progress in a notebook. Create three columns and give them a score from 1 to 10:

- Energy Level (1 = exhausted, 10 = vibrant)
- Cravings (1 = non-existent, 10 = extreme)
- Bloating (1 = calm stomach, 10 = extremely bloated)

Start to compare your ratings from week to week – they should always be improving. If your scores aren't improving after one week, try the following:

### FOR LOW ENERGY (1–4):

- Drink your morning salt water immediately upon waking (before coffee, before checking your phone).
- Add slightly more salt to your morning water.
- Increase your total daily water intake.
- Make sure you're drinking consistently throughout the day, not just chugging large amounts sporadically.

### FOR PERSISTENT CRAVINGS (7–10):

- Check you're using enough salt in your morning water (you should taste it slightly).
- Make sure you do the afternoon hydration boost immediately when the 3 p.m. slump hits.
- Ensure you're not waiting too long between the morning salt water and your first meal.

### FOR ONGOING BLOATING (7–10):

- Start with a smaller pinch of salt and gradually increase over the week.
- Try adding lemon to your morning salt water to aid digestion.
- Space your water intake more evenly throughout the day rather than drinking large amounts at once.
- Consider if you're drinking too close to meals (try leaving 30 minutes before eating).

Now that we have a stable foundation, it's time to tackle the next, most powerful metabolic switch. In the next chapter, we are going to learn how to manage your fuel. We are going to flatten your blood sugar curve and put an end to cravings for good.

**CHAPTER 2**

# THE BLOOD SUGAR SEQUENCE

The glow of the television flickered across my face, mixing with the tears tracking through my make-up. It was 11 p.m. on a Friday, and I was on the sofa, spooning ice cream straight from the tub. I wasn't even tasting it anymore, just swallowing mouthfuls robotically, trying to block out my failures. This was my ritual. Every 'good' week ended exactly like this: after five days of punishing workouts and joyless, low-calorie meals, it would all be cancelled out by one night of exhaustion, stress and a craving so powerful I felt possessed.

Maybe your Friday night looks different – maybe it's a bottle of wine while mindlessly scrolling Deliveroo, or eating half a packet of biscuits without noticing – but I bet you've had your own version of this moment: when all the 'good' choices in the week unravel in one sitting, and you're left wondering why you can't just stay strong. 'Why do I have zero willpower? Why can't I stick to "no dessert" for even one night? And why does sugar call my name like it's got me on speed-dial?'

If misinformation burned calories, you'd already be in the best shape of your life. You've been told to cut carbs as if they were a toxic ex. To treat sugar like a gateway drug. To put butter in your coffee because a guy on a podcast promised it would turn you into a 'fat-burning machine'. You've survived on joy-free diets, tried Keto, intermittent fasting and juice cleanses. And every Monday, you've begun with religious commitment, only to have the whole thing crumble by the weekend, leaving you back on the sofa wondering: *What is fundamentally wrong with me?*

You have been blaming your willpower for a problem that is about your blood sugar. The evening food-demon version of yourself? She was created by stuff that happened earlier in the day, sometimes even days before.

This chapter is going to show you how to stop this weekly mess before it even starts. It's about a simple, ridiculously easy sequence that will balance your blood sugar, switch off your cravings and put an end to that mid-afternoon energy slump for good. This isn't about restriction. It's about science. And it's the key to finally getting off the blood sugar rollercoaster and taking back control.

## PAPER FIRES VS. SLOW LOGS: WHY SOME CALORIES ARE LIARS

Before we go any further, we need to sort out one lie we've all been told: that all calories are the same.

The idea that 100 calories from an avocado and 100 calories from a biscuit are the same is the biggest lie in nutrition. Yes, they contain the same amount of *energy*. But they trigger a completely different biological and hormonal conversation in your body.

Imagine your metabolism (your body's energy-burning system) is a fireplace. Consuming 100 calories from a biscuit – which is mostly refined carbohydrates and sugar – is like throwing a piece of paper on the fire. You get a huge, hot, fast flame (i.e. a massive energy spike) that dies out in 60 seconds, leaving you with nothing but ash and in need of more fuel (i.e. a blood sugar crash and intense cravings). But eating 100 calories from an avocado – mostly healthy fats and fibre – is like putting a dense, heavy log on the fire. It catches slowly and burns with a steady, consistent, reliable heat for hours, providing stable, long-lasting energy.

When you eat that biscuit, your body releases insulin – that's the hormone that creates the dramatic spike and crash – to deal with the sugar rush. The avocado barely triggers insulin at all, keeping your energy steady. The difference in this hormonal response is the main reason why the 100 calories from the avocado and the 100 calories from the biscuit are not the same.

And there's another reveal about the 'all calories are equal' lie. It's not just about the hormonal signal a food sends; it's also about the metabolic effort needed to digest and process it. Foods rich in protein and fibre are not just 'slow logs' for your blood sugar; they are also metabolically 'expensive', forcing your body to burn more calories just to access their energy. Basically, your body has to work harder to process some foods than others – a scientific concept called the thermic effect of food (TEF).

TEF is essentially the energy 'cost' of digestion. Think of it like a tax. When you eat, your body must expend energy to break down, absorb and process the nutrients from that food. Different types of food are taxed at different rates, depending on which macronutrients they mainly contain.

Macronutrients are simply the three main building blocks of all food: protein, carbohydrates and fats. Protein has the highest tax because your body burns about 30 per cent of protein calories just trying to break it down. So, from 100 calories of chicken, you're only getting about 70 calories' worth of actual energy.

Carbohydrates have a medium tax rate, at around 5 to 10 per cent. Fat is the easiest for your body to process and has the lowest tax rate, at just 0 to 3 per cent.

Let's look at our avocado versus our biscuit through this lens. The biscuit is mostly carbs and fat, the two most easily processed macronutrients. Your body barely breaks a sweat digesting it. The 100 calories you eat is effectively 100 calories of available energy. The avocado, on the other hand, contains fibre, fat and a little bit of protein. Your body must work significantly harder to break it down and extract the energy.

For years, you've been throwing wads of paper onto your metabolic fire – think high-in-refined-carbs cereal for breakfast, a high-in-refined-carbs sandwich for lunch – and then wondering why you feel exhausted and ravenous a few hours later.

The craving-control sequence we are going to come to is about learning to put the protective logs on the fire *first*. This sequence is not just a clever physical hack to slow down digestion; it's also a powerful hormonal strategy. The order in which you eat sends a direct instruction to your gut to release a cascade of hormones that fundamentally change how you experience a meal.

The most important of these hormones is called GLP-1 (glucagon-like peptide-1). You can think of GLP-1 as your body's own natural Ozempic. It's an incredibly intelligent hormone released from the cells of your gut in response to food, and it does two truly magical things. First, it travels to your brain and signals a feeling of fullness and satisfaction. Second, it travels to your pancreas and gives it a gentle, preparatory nudge, saying, 'Get ready, some carbohydrates are on their way, so let's prepare a calm, measured insulin response.'

Here's the secret: different foods trigger the release of GLP-1 at different speeds. Protein and fat are powerful GLP-1 stimulators. When you eat your vegetables (fibre) and your protein and fat *before* your carbohydrates, you are sending out an early warning signal. You are stimulating a strong, early release of this amazing satiety hormone. The result? By the time you get to the starchy or sugary part of your meal, your brain is already receiving signals that you are feeling full. This makes you far less likely to overeat the carbohydrate portion of the meal. You feel satisfied with a smaller amount. On top of that, your pancreas is already prepped and ready, so the insulin response it produces is more controlled and efficient, rather than being a panicked surge.

So, the sequence isn't just about managing the traffic on the road. It's like sending a brilliant traffic cop (GLP-1) ahead to calmly direct busy streets, giving the nod to who moves when and ensuring everything flows smoothly from a hormonal perspective. It's an internal chemical conversation, and by eating your food in the right order, you are speaking your body's language.

## GLUCOSE SPIKE 101: WHAT'S REALLY HAPPENING INSIDE YOUR BODY

You've probably heard the term 'glucose spike' or 'blood sugar spike' thrown around by health influencers or in articles you've read. But what does that actually *mean*? What is physically happening inside your body when you eat that bowl of cereal or that sandwich for lunch? And why does it matter so much?

Let's have a quick tour of the biological rollercoaster you've been riding every day without even knowing it.

### THE CLIMB

When you eat a meal that's mostly 'paper fire' carbohydrates, your digestive system breaks them down quickly into their simplest form: glucose. This glucose floods your bloodstream. Imagine all the carriages of a rollercoaster being winched up that first steep hill very, very quickly. *Click, click, click, click, click.* This is the 'spike'. It's a rapid, steep increase in the amount of sugar circulating in your blood.

## THE PEAK (THE PROBLEM)

At the top of the hill, your body panics. All the glucose in the bloodstream is toxic if it stays there for too long. So, your pancreas releases a massive surge of insulin – think of it as the rollercoaster's emergency braking system kicking in to counteract its dangerous high speed.

## THE PLUNGE (THE PART YOU FEEL)

Here's the problem: the emergency brakes are so powerful they don't just slow the rollercoaster down, they send it hurtling down the other side of the hill even faster than before. Your blood sugar doesn't level out, coming back to normal; instead, it crashes far below where it started. The rollercoaster overshoots the terminus and plunges into a deep valley.

This is the 'crash'. The moment that defines so much of your daily energy struggle.

This crash is what you experience as:

- The 3 p.m. energy slump that feels like you've been drugged.
- The sudden brain fog when you can't seem to string a sentence together.
- The shaky, irritable, almost murderous feeling known as 'hanger'.
- The intense, uncontrollable craving for more sugar or carbs, which is your brain's desperate attempt to get the rollercoaster back up the hill again.

## THE HIDDEN DAMAGE

This chaos isn't just annoying, it's doing damage. Every time you go on one of these blood sugar rollercoasters, it's like setting off a tiny earthquake in your body. It creates inflammation, pumps out stress hormones like cortisol (which tells your body to store belly fat) and, over time, your cells start getting 'deaf' to insulin's signals. That's how you end up with insulin resistance.

For years, you've been beating yourself up about your personality flaws: 'I'm just not a morning person', 'I've got zero willpower in the afternoon'. But it's not your character traits; it's just biology doing what it's supposed to do when you feed it the wrong fuel at the wrong time.

The good news is that you can turn this erratic rollercoaster into a gentle, rolling ride. No more dramatic spikes and crashes. It all starts with something dead simple: the order in which you eat your food.

## THE SYSTEM: THE CRAVING-CONTROL SEQUENCE

So, you understand why your body treats different foods so differently – why that biscuit creates chaos while the avocado keeps things steady. You know about the fireplace effect, the hormonal signals, and how much energy different foods cost to process. We understand what's happening inside our bodies; we can look at how we can balance out the spikes and crashes. The question is: what do you actually DO with this knowledge?

The science on this is clear. Studies have shown that by simply changing the order in which you eat the components of your meal, you can slash the subsequent glucose spike by up to 73 per cent.[2] This is the craving-control sequence. It is your new, non-negotiable rule for breakfast, lunch and dinner.

Now, I know what you're thinking; 'What if I can't always follow this sequence perfectly?' Life happens. Sometimes you'll grab a sandwich on the go, or find yourself at a restaurant where the sequence gets muddled. That's completely normal. Here's the thing: this sequence is your craving-control foundation. When you follow it, you'll notice your afternoon energy crashes disappear and your evening food cravings settle down. When life gets chaotic and you can't follow it perfectly, that's fine – just come back to it at your next meal. The goal isn't perfection: it's giving you a tool that works. Think of it as your reliable backup plan that you can return to whenever you feel those old patterns of spikes and crashes creeping back in.

## STEP 1: FIBRE FIRST

**The how:** Start with your fibre sources first – vegetables, salads, beans and pulses: the side salad, the broccoli, the lentils, the chickpeas, whatever high-fibre foods you've chosen. Eat these before you touch anything else.

**The why:** The fibre creates a gel-like mesh in your gut that acts like a sieve, slowing down how fast any sugar from carbs is absorbed later.

## STEP 2: PROTEIN AND FATS SECOND

**The how:** After your fibre sources, eat your protein and fat source: the eggs, the chicken, the salmon, the yogurt, the tofu.

**The why:** Protein and fat also put the brakes on digestion and signal the release of hormones that tell your brain, 'We're getting full now.'

## STEP 3: CARBS LAST

**The how:** Finally, you eat your starches and sugars. The potatoes, the rice, the pasta, the bread.

**The why:** By now you've built a sturdy buffer system. Instead of those carbs hitting your bloodstream like a sugar bomb, they'll trickle in nice and gently. No chaos, just steady energy.

## THE TRAFFIC JAM

Back to our bloodstream road analogy. Eating carbs first is like opening a slip road and letting 500 cars flood onto an empty motorway all at once. It causes a massive traffic jam (a glucose spike), requiring an emergency intervention (insulin). Eating in the correct order is like having a clever traffic management system. The vegetables are the traffic cones; the protein and fat are the traffic lights. The same 500 cars get onto the motorway, but they do it in a calm, orderly fashion. This one simple change is the difference between a steady flow of energy and a chaotic, craving-inducing traffic jam in your body.

## THE HORMONAL HANGOVER: THE REAL COST OF A BLOOD SUGAR SPIKE

The effect of the traffic jam in your body isn't just obvious at the time; it turns into what I call the 'hormonal hangover', which can cause damage for at least the next 24 hours.

When you have a massive glucose spike, your pancreas releases a huge surge of insulin to deal with it. About two hours afterwards, your blood sugar levels plummet, precipitating a biological crisis. Your body perceives this as a threat and releases the stress hormones – cortisol and adrenaline – to bring your blood sugar back up.

Now you're not just dealing with low blood sugar; you're also marinating in stress hormones. This is why you feel shaky, irritable and anxious after a sugar crash. It's a physiological stress response. This cortisol spike then signals to your body to store fat (especially around your middle), it disrupts your sleep later that night, and it sets you up for even more intense cravings the next day.

A single, poorly balanced meal can create a negative hormonal ripple effect that lasts for a full 24 hours.

> **AMELIA'S STORY**
>
> Graphic designer Amelia worked from home. Her biggest complaint was the 3 p.m. wall. 'It's like clockwork,' she told me. 'I'll have a healthy lunch, like a chicken sandwich, and by 3 o'clock, I can't keep my eyes open. My brain just switches off, and the only thing I can think about is raiding the kids' snack cupboard.'
>
> Her 'healthy' lunch was sliced roasted chicken between two thick slices of buttered bread. While this sounds balanced, the problem was that the bread was dominating the meal: two large slices created a massive carb load that overwhelmed the smaller amount of protein.
>
> I didn't change what she was eating. I just changed the order. Her new, deconstructed lunch looked like this:
>
> - **Step 1:** Start with a big side salad (lettuce, tomatoes, cucumber).
> - **Step 2:** Next, eat the sliced chicken.
> - **Step 3:** Finally, eat the buttered bread slices.
>
> Three days later, I got a message. 'This is so weird. It's 4 p.m., and I'm not tired. At all. I'm not even *thinking* about the snack cupboard.'

Now, before you panic about having to deconstruct everything, you don't have to. If it really feels too odd, then do a gentler version. The principle is simple: just get substantial fibre and protein in before the bread. You could just as easily:

- Have a proper side salad with your sandwich, eating the salad first.
- Start with raw veggies and hummus, then eat your sandwich.
- Eat the filling of your sandwich, then your salad, finishing with the bread.

## THE PROTEIN-PACKED BREAKFAST MASTERCLASS: YOUR MOST IMPORTANT MEAL

Remember your morning salt water? That was step one of setting yourself up for success. Step two is equally crucial; if there is one eating habit that will change your life more than any other, it is this:

Start your day with protein.

The first meal of the day sets your metabolic tone and blood sugar baseline for the next 24 hours. Starting with a carb-heavy meal – cereal, toast, a croissant, 'healthy' granola, a fruit-only smoothie – is like starting your day by setting a giant bonfire of paper on fire. It guarantees a mid-morning crash and a day spent on a chaotic energy rollercoaster.

Your breakfast must be built around protein and healthy fats. Aim for 25 to 35 grams of protein.

**The why:** A protein-first breakfast does three magical things. It has a minimal impact on your blood sugar, providing a stable foundation and thereby helping to regulate your appetite hormones for the rest of the day, making you less likely to crave sugar in the afternoon. It is also highly satiating, keeping you full and focused for hours. But the real magic of a protein-first breakfast goes even deeper than blood sugar. It fundamentally changes your brain chemistry, particularly your relationship with a powerful neurotransmitter called dopamine.

Dopamine is often called the 'pleasure chemical', but it's more like your motivation system – it gets you excited about achieving stuff. Protein contains amino acids that your brain needs to make dopamine. Starting your day with protein can help to keep your mood and focus more stable, rather than constantly chasing quick hits of satisfaction from sugar or other instant rewards.

It's not magic, but it's one part of keeping your brain chemistry working with you instead of against you.

Starting your day with a sugar bomb like cereal or pastries gives you a quick energy high, but it crashes fast. It destabilises your brain's entire reward system. When your blood sugar drops, you're more likely to crave another quick fix – more sugar, or even distractions like scrolling on your phone. Protein-based breakfasts keep your energy more stable. It's about achieving a steady fuel versus the rollercoaster.

Protein at the beginning of the day doesn't just balance your blood sugar, it balances your brain. You are preparing yourself for a day of calm, focused energy, rather than a frantic, desperate search for your next fix.

## YOUR BREAKFAST BLUEPRINT

*25–35g protein breakfast examples*
- 3 scrambled eggs (18g) + 2 slices ham (8g) + half an avocado = 26g
- 150g Greek yogurt + handful nuts (6g) + a handful of berries = 26g
- 2-egg omelette (12g) + cheese (8g) + smoked salmon (10g) = 30g
- Protein smoothie: 1 scoop protein powder (25g) + milk (8g) = 33g

### The 5-minute scramble

4 eggs (24g protein) scrambled with a handful of spinach, raw or cooked, and 30g of cheddar cheese (8g protein). Total roughly 32g protein.

### The protein yogurt bowl

150g Greek yogurt (15g protein) mixed with a scoop of protein powder (25g protein), topped with a handful of berries and 2 tablespoons of mixed nuts (4g protein). Total: 44g protein (perfect for post-workout or particularly busy days when you need extra fuel).

### The savoury cottage cheese bowl

A pot of cottage cheese (25g protein) topped with sliced tomatoes, cucumber, olive oil and a sprinkle of seasoning. Add 2 tablespoons of nuts or seeds (4g protein). Total roughly 30g protein.

### The speedy smoothie

A high-quality protein powder (25g protein), a tablespoon of almond butter (4g protein), a handful of spinach and unsweetened almond milk. (Notice: build smoothies around protein, not just fruit.) Total roughly 29g protein.

And if you can't handle 4 eggs? Here are some alternatives that hit the same protein target:

- 3 eggs + extra cheese: 3 eggs (18g) + 45g cheddar (11g) = 29g protein
- 3 eggs + bacon: 3 eggs (18g) + 2 strips bacon (6g) + cheese (7g) = 31g protein
- 2 eggs + Greek yogurt: 2 eggs (12g) + 150g Greek yogurt (15g) + cheese (7g) = 34g protein

Again, the goal is 25–35g protein at breakfast – find what works for your appetite and preferences.

## THE CRASH-PROOF SNACK MATRIX

Snacking isn't a crime, but mindless snacking on carbohydrates alone will put you back on the blood sugar rollercoaster. Follow this simple rule:

Never let a carb go solo – always give it a mate, be it protein or fat.

Yes, you did just read that right: this approach actually encourages you to eat more, not less. Unlike restrictive diets that leave you hungry and deprived, this method works by nourishing your body properly. You're not cutting calories or eliminating food groups – you're simply pairing foods strategically to keep your blood sugar stable. And the result? Better health, natural weight loss and enjoying your food. This isn't about following another dull diet, it's about making a sustainable lifestyle change that your body will thank you for.

| Choose a carb (the energy) | Pair with a 'protector' (the brakes) |
| --- | --- |
| An apple | A tablespoon of almond butter or a slice of cheese |
| A handful of berries | A small pot of full-fat Greek yogurt |
| 2–3 rice cakes | Sliced avocado or a few slices of turkey |
| A banana | A handful of walnuts or a hard-boiled egg |
| A square of dark chocolate | A small handful of almonds |

And then, of course, there are the advertising lies, the misunderstandings, the family beliefs ... all the things you thought you knew about 'healthy' foods but didn't know to check up on.

## BUSTING THE 'HEALTHY' FOOD MYTHS

### 'What about my "healthy" granola?'
Turn the packet around and look at the sugar content. Most commercial granolas are biscuit crumbs in a fancy box. If you love it, use it as a small 'sprinkle' on top of a high-protein Greek yogurt bowl, not as the main event.

### 'Are juice cleanses a good way to reset?'
A juice cleanse is just a multi-day sugar bomb that spikes your insulin, contains zero fibre or protein, and puts your body under massive stress. The weight you lose is almost entirely water and muscle. So, no, not a good way to reset!

### 'I start every day with a big fruit smoothie. Isn't that good for me?'
A smoothie that is just fruit and a liquid base is a fast track to a blood sugar crash. To make a smoothie work for you, it must be built like a balanced meal: start with a scoop of protein powder, add a tablespoon of fat (like avocado or nut butter), add a fist of greens (like spinach) and *then* add a small, cupped handful of fruit for flavour.

## TOP BLOOD SUGAR HACKS

### THE COOLING TRICK (RESISTANT STARCH)

Cook your potatoes and rice, then stick them in the fridge. When you eat them cold (think potato salad or leftover rice), some of the starch changes into resistant starch (i.e. it resists digestion), which is much gentler on your blood sugar.

But here's where it gets interesting – this resistant starch and other fibres don't just help your blood sugar. They're also brilliant news for the good bacteria living in your gut. Think of your gut bacteria as your own little internal factory. When you feed them the right stuff (like these fibres), they churn out some rather amazing compounds for you – short-chain fatty acids that help reduce inflammation, keep your gut lining healthy and even improve your cells' response to insulin. Some benefits include:

- **Healing your gut:** When fibre reaches your gut, your healthy bacteria produce a compound called butyrate (think of it as food for your gut lining). This feeds the cells lining your gut, keeping everything in good nick and reducing inflammation effects.
- **Reducing inflammation:** These compounds help to decrease inflammation throughout your body, which is brilliant for your overall health.
- **Improving insulin sensitivity:** Here's the clever bit – these gut compounds can make your cells more responsive to insulin. They help your cells listen better to insulin's signals.

This all creates a positive cycle. Eating more fibre makes your gut healthier. A healthier gut produces more of these good compounds. And those compounds help you handle blood sugar better. Everything's connected. By feeding your gut bacteria with the right stuff, once again you're helping to regulate that blood sugar rollercoaster.

More good news, too: you don't have to eat these foods cold: research shows that resistant starch levels remain elevated after reheating foods that have previously been cooled. Cook your rice, potatoes or pasta, cool them in the fridge overnight, then reheat and enjoy – you'll still get the blood sugar benefits. In fact, with pasta, reheating after cooling gives even better results than eating it cold.

## A NOTE FOR SHIFT WORKERS

Your body clock is tied to your first meal. Your 'breakfast' is whatever meal you eat when you wake up, even if it's at 8 p.m. Start your 'day' with a high-protein meal and apply the craving-control sequence to your other meals relative to your own schedule.

# WORKING WITH YOUR CYCLE

Your insulin sensitivity naturally fluctuates throughout your menstrual cycle. It's generally at its best in the first half (the follicular phase) and can dip in the week before your period (the luteal phase). This is why you crave carbs before your period! Don't fight it; work with it. Strategically, increasing your intake of smart, slow carbs (like sweet potatoes and quinoa) in that pre-menstrual week can help to support progesterone production, boost serotonin and mitigate PMS-driven cravings. If you struggle with insulin sensitivity, having your main carb portion with your evening meal rather than at lunch can sometimes improve sleep and hormonal balance.

> **THE MONTHLY MAP: YOUR FOUR INNER SEASONS**
>
> Think of your monthly cycle as having four distinct 'inner seasons'. Each season has a unique hormonal climate that directly influences your energy, your mood, your appetite and even your creativity. Learning to identify which season you're in is the first step to working *with* your body, not against it.

## THE BLOOD SUGAR SEQUENCE

*The follicular phase (your inner spring)*

- **When:** This phase starts after your period ends and lasts until you ovulate. This could be anywhere from 7 to 14 days depending on your individual cycle length.
- **What's happening:** After your period, the hormone oestrogen begins a steady climb. Think of it as the sun starting to come out after a long winter, warming everything up and bringing new life.
- **How you might feel:** Your energy and optimism start to build. Your brain feels clearer and sharper. You're generally more resilient to stress, your appetite is stable and manageable. This is a time of renewal and possibility.
- **The opportunity:** This is the perfect time to start something new. Kick off a new project at work, try a more challenging workout or plan a social get-together. Your body is primed for action and growth.

*The ovulatory phase (your inner summer)*

- **When:** A short, vibrant window in the middle of your cycle, lasting 2 to 4 days (around day 14 in a 28-day cycle).
- **What's happening:** Oestrogen hits its peak, and you experience a small, helpful surge of testosterone. This is your biological prime time.
- **How you might feel:** You are at your peak. Your energy is at its highest, you feel more confident. You might notice you look and feel your best during this phase. Communication is easier.
- **The opportunity:** Channel this peak energy! Schedule that important meeting or presentation. Go on that date. Tackle your most demanding workout of the month. Say yes to social plans. This is your season to shine.

### *The luteal phase (your inner autumn)*

- **When:** This is the longest phase, lasting from after ovulation until your period begins (roughly days 15 to 28).
- **What's happening:** The hormone progesterone rises to take centre stage. Progesterone is a calming, nesting hormone. Then, in the final week before your period, both oestrogen and progesterone take a nosedive. This sudden drop is what triggers PMS symptoms.
- **How you might feel:** Energy starts to wane. You might feel more inward, anxious or easily irritated. This is when cravings for carbs and comfort foods are a genuine biological reality, not a character flaw. Your body becomes more sensitive to stress, and it's calling out for comfort and fuel.
- **The opportunity:** This is not the time to white-knuckle your way through, forcing yourself through with sheer willpower and determination. This is the season for self-compassion. Shift your focus from high-intensity to nurturing activities. Think gentle walks instead of sprints. Think nourishing, warm foods.

### *The menstrual phase (your inner winter)*

- **When:** The first few days of your bleed (roughly days 1 to 5).
- **What's happening:** Both oestrogen and progesterone are at their lowest point. Your body is directing a huge amount of energy towards shedding the uterine lining.
- **How you might feel:** Tired, withdrawn and potentially crampy or sore. Your social battery might be completely empty. You may feel the need to retreat and be alone.
- **The opportunity:** Give yourself permission to rest. This is your body's built-in time for hibernation and recovery. Pushing through with intense workouts and a packed

schedule now will only steal energy from your upcoming 'Spring'. Prioritise sleep, gentle movement, like stretching, and warm, easily digestible foods, like soups and stews.

Knowing your inner seasons is step one. Step two is having simple, powerful levers you can pull to make the more difficult seasons easier.

### Lever 1: Anchor yourself with a protein minimum

On days when cravings feel intense and your appetite seems like a bottomless pit, your first instinct might be to restrict. I want you to do the opposite: *add*.

Just ask yourself at each meal, 'Where is my anchor of at least 25 to 30 grams of protein?' This could be a chicken breast, a piece of fish, a scoop of protein powder in a smoothie, a hearty serving of Greek yogurt or cottage cheese, or a tofu scramble.

You will be amazed at how often the craving is quieted simply by giving your body the actual, substantial fuel it was asking for.

### Lever 2: Use carbs strategically for calm and sleep

In the week or two before your period, your levels of the feel-good brain chemical, serotonin, naturally dip. Your brain knows a shortcut to make more serotonin: carbohydrates. Fighting this need is a losing battle. So, let's be strategic.

A serving of smart carbs in the evening can help lower the stress hormone cortisol and support the production of serotonin. Serotonin is a precursor to melatonin, the hormone that helps you fall asleep and stay asleep, and a good night's sleep is infinitely more important for your metabolism and next-day willpower than avoiding sweet potato. This isn't about a free-for-all on pizza and cake. It's a deliberate choice: a small baked sweet potato, a cup of butternut squash, a serving of brown rice or quinoa, or even a piece of fruit.

# YOUR SECOND ACTION PLAN: THE BLOOD SUGAR RESET

**The mindset shift:** This isn't about restriction – it's about foundation. You're not depriving yourself of anything, you're giving yourself the fuel that actually works.

**The goal:** Collect concrete proof of how this simple sequence change makes you feel.

## 1: SWAP THE ORDER

**The task:** Change the order in which you eat your food: fibre first, protein/fats second, carbs last.

- Start your day with a savoury, high-protein breakfast.
- Always pair carbs with protein or fat.

## 2: THE 3-DAY EXPERIMENT

**The practice:** For the next three days, for your lunch and dinner, you will follow the craving-control sequence to the letter: fibre first, protein/fats second, and carbs last.

**The data collection:** At the end of each day, track two things in a notebook, with a score from 1 to 10.

- 3 p.m. energy level (1 = zombie, 10 = superhero)
- Evening craving intensity (1 = couldn't care less about snacks, 10 = raiding the cupboards)

If you want to really motor, swap your usual breakfast for one of the high-protein options from the breakfast blueprint on page 45.

You now have the key to calm days. By stabilising your blood sugar, you are creating a foundation of stable energy. However, a calm day often hinges on a restful night. In the next chapter, we're going to explore how to repay your energy debts and turn your sleep into your secret, fat-burning weapon.

# CHAPTER 3
# RECLAIMING THE NIGHT – THE VALUE OF SLEEP

You've been misled about what it takes to change your body. You've been told that success means running yourself into the ground; that real progress only happens when you're smashing yourself in the gym, spending hours meal-prepping like you're going to war and treating your body like it's the problem that needs fixing. Sleep? That's something lazy people do when they should be working harder.

And you treat it just like a luxury you can't afford. You're answering emails at 11 p.m., scrolling Instagram in bed, then dragging yourself up at 5 a.m. for a workout. You tell yourself this is what commitment looks like, that if you push harder during the day it'll make up for the rubbish sleep at night.

What if I told you that this is the single biggest mistake you are making? What if I told you that you don't need more discipline during the day but deeper sleep at night? What if I told you that eight hours spent in bed are not an inconvenience, but are, in fact, the most potent, powerful and productive fat-burning, muscle-building and hormone-balancing gift you have?

This chapter is about reframing sleep from a passive dead time when nothing is achieved, into your ultimate advantage. I am going to show you how a few simple tweaks to your evening routine can switch on your body's most powerful repair and fat-loss machinery, making every other healthy choice during the day much more effective.

It's time to stop seeing sleep as a luxury and to start treating it like the superpower it is.

## THE SCIENCE: MEET YOUR BRAIN'S NIGHT SHIFT

While you are unconscious, your body is anything but. The moment you hit deep sleep, it's like a maintenance crew clocks on for the night shift. They're doing all the repair work you don't have time for during the day – fixing muscles, sorting out hormones and keeping everything running smoothly. Skip sleep and it's like expecting a city to function without all the street cleaners and repair crews. Eventually, everything falls apart.

Let's meet the key members of your overnight crew.

### THE HORMONE RE-BALANCERS: GHRELIN AND LEPTIN

You've likely experienced this: after a bad night's sleep, you wake up feeling not just tired, but ravenous. Your cravings for sugar and carbs are through the roof, and no matter what you eat, you can't seem to feel full. This isn't a failure of your willpower; it's your sleep-deprived brain messing with your hormones.

Your appetite is controlled by two key hormones that work like a see-saw:

- **Ghrelin (the 'go' hormone):** Produced in your stomach, it sends a powerful signal to your brain that says, 'GO! EAT! I'M HUNGRY!'

- **Leptin (the 'stop' hormone):** This is the sensible one. It's produced by your fat cells and sends a signal to your brain that says, 'STOP! We're full and satisfied. You can put the fork down now.'

During a night of deep, restorative sleep, your body carefully recalibrates this see-saw. It suppresses ghrelin and sensitises your brain to leptin, setting you up for a day of normal, manageable hunger and clear fullness signals. When you get a poor night's sleep, the see-saw is completely thrown out of whack. Studies have shown that even one night of insufficient or no sleep can raise ghrelin (the hunger hormone) by around 20–25 per cent in healthy people, while leptin (the satiety hormone) may decrease, though not always to a statistically significant degree.[3] The result? You wake up with the ghrelin (think 'the ghrelin gremlin' – demanding food) while sensible leptin is locked in a soundproof room. As a result, you are hormonally programmed to be hungrier, to crave high-calorie, sugary foods and to feel less full, no matter what you eat. You are fighting a chemical battle you cannot win.

A good night's sleep is the most effective appetite suppressant you can take.

## THE FAT-BURNING FOREMAN: HUMAN GROWTH HORMONE

Deep sleep isn't just resting time, it's when your body is busy rebuilding itself. This is when you experience a hit of growth hormone, which acts like your body's night manager. During this phase, your pituitary gland releases a huge dose of human growth hormone (HGH).

This hormone oversees two crucial projects while you're sleeping.

- **Repairs and builds muscle:** HGH is the primary driver of muscle protein synthesis. It takes the protein you've eaten and uses it to repair the microscopic tears in your muscles, building them back stronger and denser. Since muscle tissue burns more calories than fat tissue – even at rest – this directly increases your metabolic rate (the speed at which your body burns calories throughout the day).
- **Burns fat for fuel:** While it's building muscle, HGH also signals to your fat cells to release stored fatty acids into the bloodstream to be used for energy. It flips your body into its primary fat-burning state.

Here's the catch: most of this happens in our first few hours of proper deep sleep. Cut your sleep short or keep waking up, and you're telling your night manager to go home early. No repairs happen; no fat gets burned.

## THE BRAIN'S STREET SWEEPER: THE GLYMPHATIC SYSTEM

Have you ever experienced 'brain fog' after a bad night's sleep? That feeling of being slow, fuzzy and unable to think clearly? That's not just tiredness; that's your brain sitting in yesterday's mess because the night shift cleaners didn't turn up.

Think about it this way. Every night while you're asleep, your brain resembles a city centre at 3 a.m., with power washers going full blast cleaning the streets. The spaces between your brain cells – and I'm talking proper microscopic gaps here – get bigger during deep sleep. Fluid comes rushing through like it's hosing down the pavements, collecting all the metabolic rubbish your brain produced during the day and flushing it out. Scientists call it the glymphatic system, but I just think of it as your brain's cleaning crew working the night shift.

And here's the part that'll really blow your mind: the main rubbish it's clearing out is a protein called beta-amyloid. The same stuff that builds up in people's brains with Alzheimer's.

So, when you're surviving on four hours' sleep thinking you're being productive, you're really just leaving toxic waste sitting in your brain. Mental, right?

And as for the 'I'm just a bad sleeper' lie we tell ourselves? I swear, if I had a pound for every woman who's told me 'I've always been a terrible sleeper, it's just who I am,' I could probably retire to a villa in Spain tomorrow.

Let's break that phrase down ...

### HANNAH'S STORY

Hannah is 35 years old, a marketing director, and an absolute perfectionist when it comes to her nutrition and training. She was hitting her workouts three times a week, had her meal prep sorted, but felt like death warmed up most days.

'I've just always been this way,' she told me, a resigned exhaustion in her voice. 'It takes me ages to fall asleep because my brain won't switch off, and then I wake up at 3 a.m. every single night, my heart pounding, and I lie there for hours worrying about my to-do list.'

Hannah has a classic case of being wired-but-exhausted. That horrible, buzzy feeling in the evening when your cortisol's through the roof, but then waking up feeling like you've been hit by a truck.

Hannah was convinced she was just broken, born with dodgy sleep genes or similar. But when I looked at what she was doing before bed it was no wonder she couldn't sleep.

9 p.m. Still answering work emails on her laptop. In bed. Blue light blazing straight into her eyeballs.

> 9.30 p.m. 'Wind-down time' – aka scrolling Instagram looking at everyone else's highlight reels while her brain was becoming more wired by the second.
>
> 10 p.m. Healthy snack time! A nice piece of fruit. But also a sugar bomb right when her body's trying to power down for the night.

And Hannah wondered why she couldn't sleep!

Similar to a lot of us, Hannah had fallen into a modern-day trap. She wasn't sending 'time for bed' signals to her body, she was sending 'WAKE UP' signals, and then getting frustrated when her biology did exactly what she'd asked it to do.

Hannah's transformation didn't come from some fancy sleep supplement or a £200 silk pillowcase. It came from one simple realisation: she wasn't a bad sleeper, she just had a negative evening routine.

We created what I call the 'switch-off hour'. Nothing revolutionary: just based around the basic biology that respects how your body works.

### THE 'SWITCH-OFF HOUR' PROTOCOL

**60 minutes before bed**

- Laptop gets shut and put in another room (not just closed – gone).
- Phone goes on airplane mode or gets plugged in somewhere you can't reach it from bed.
- No sugar, no stimulants, no 'healthy' fruit snacks that spike your blood sugar.

> - Dim the lights – we're talking proper cave-like vibes.
> - Do something genuinely relaxing: read a book, have a bath, listen to a podcast about something mind-numbing.

Within two weeks, Hannah was sleeping through the night. Her afternoon cravings disappeared. She started seeing results from her workouts because her body could finally recover properly at night.

She didn't fix herself – she just fixed her evenings.

The mad part? She thought she'd tried everything. Turns out she'd never tried the one thing that matters: treating sleep like the biological necessity it is, instead of something that should just happen automatically.

Your brain needs its night shift cleaners. Give them a chance to do their job and notice how different you feel when you wake up with a properly 'clean' mind instead of yesterday's rubbish cluttering up your head.

## THE SYSTEM: THE UNBREAKABLE SLEEP PROTOCOL

This is not about chasing a perfect eight hours. It's about creating the ideal conditions for your body to get the deep, restorative sleep it needs, whatever your schedule. This is your 'power-down hour' checklist.

### 1. LIGHT CONTROL: TURNING YOUR HOUSE INTO A COSY CAVE

**The why:** Your brain automatically thinks that artificial light = daytime = stay awake. Every bright light you're staring at is like shouting 'MORNING TIME!' at your sleep hormones.

**The protocol:**
- **Kill the big lights:** Turn off those horrible overhead spotlights. Use table lamps with warm bulbs instead – think pub lighting, not operating theatre.
- **Activate night mode:** All devices go on night mode. Blue light (e.g. screen light) is light-wave caffeine for your eyeballs.
- **If you absolutely must work late:** Get some blue light-blocking glasses. They look a bit wild but they work.

> **THE PARTNER PROBLEM TWEAK**
>
> Sharing a bed with someone who scrolls at full brightness is like trying to sleep next to a lighthouse; it gets tricky when your other half thinks bedtime means catching up on TikTok with the screen brightness set to 'surface of the sun'.
>
> Don't become the sleep police – nobody likes that person. Instead, try this: 'I've been reading about how light affects sleep and energy. Fancy trying a "no phones in bed" experiment with me for a week? Just to see if we both feel better?'
>
> Frame it as something you're doing together, not something they're doing wrong. And if they're not having it? Invest in a decent silk eye mask. Your sleep is non-negotiable, even if theirs isn't.

## 2. TEMPERATURE CONTROL: CHANNEL YOUR INNER POLAR BEAR

**The why:** Your body's core temperature naturally needs to drop by a couple of degrees to get into proper deep sleep. A bedroom that is too warm is one of the most common and overlooked sleep-disruptors.

**The protocol:**
- Aim to make your bedroom cool, dark and quiet, like a cave. The ideal temperature for sleep is surprisingly cool, around 18 to 20°C (65 to 68°F).
- A warm bath or shower an hour before bed can help. It raises your body temperature temporarily, and the subsequent rapid cool-down as you get out is a powerful signal to your brain that it's time to sleep.

### 3. THE CAFFEINE CURFEW: RESPECT THE SCIENCE, NOT YOUR FEELINGS

**The why:** Caffeine has a half-life of about 5 to 6 hours. This means that if you have a coffee at 3 p.m., half of that caffeine is *still* circulating in your system at 8 or 9 p.m. Even if you don't 'feel' the effects, it's quietly sabotaging your deep sleep without you realising.

**The protocol:** Hard cut-off: After lunch, about 2 p.m., you're done with caffeine. Switch to decaf or herbal teas instead. Yes, this includes that 'tiny' afternoon coffee: **half the caffeine is still half the caffeine.**

### 4. THE BRAIN DUMP: GET THE WORRIES OUT OF YOUR HEAD

**The why:** You know when you wake up at 3 a.m. and your mind is in overdrive, thinking about everything you need to do? That's your brain using the quiet to remind you about all the unfinished business floating around in your head.

**The protocol:** 30 minutes before bed, get a notebook (not your phone) and brain dump everything – tomorrow's to-do list, that email you forgot to send, whatever you're worrying about. Think of it like this: you're closing all the tabs on your mental browser. Once it's written down, your brain can stop trying to remember it.

None of this is revolutionary. It's just basic sleep hygiene, and it works if you follow the protocols.

Try all four protocols in the system for a week and tell me you don't feel like a different person. Or don't – but then don't complain when you're still waking up feeling like you've been hit by a truck.

## EVENING FUEL: HOW TO EAT YOUR WAY TO BETTER SLEEP

We've sorted out your lighting and temperature, but what about the stuff you're putting in your mouth before bed? Because here's the thing – what you eat (and when), can be the difference between sleeping like a baby or lying there staring at the ceiling counting sheep until 3 a.m.

### FOOD FOR SLEEP: THE 'SLEEPY CARB' AND YOUR MAGNESIUM ALLY

**The strategic evening carb:** I know, I know – everything you've heard about carbs says to avoid them at night. But this is an example of where the fitness industry gets it wrong again.

**Why evening carbs can help:** Your body has a clever system helping carbs to shuttle an amino acid called tryptophan into your brain, which then converts it into serotonin (the happy, calm hormone). This then finally becomes melatonin (your useful sleep hormone). It's like a biological assembly line that ends with you asleep.

**What to eat:**
- Three tablespoons of sweet potato.
- Some quinoa with your dinner.
- A handful of berries after your meal.
- Essentially, smart carbs that won't spike your blood sugar like a rocket.

**Important bit:** This shouldn't give you permission to demolish a bowl of pasta at 9 p.m. We're talking strategic, small amounts that work *with* your biology, not against it.

**The magnesium game-changer:** this is one of the few supplements I recommend to most people, because often we are walking around deficient in magnesium without realising it. And of the various magnesium products out there, magnesium glycinate is your best friend.

**Why magnesium glycinate specifically:**
- It's the ultimate chill-out mineral for your nervous system.
- The 'glycinate' form gets absorbed properly (unlike the cheap stuff that just goes straight through you).
- It tells your brain and muscles to relax.

**How to use it:** Take it about an hour before bed, because it needs time to get into your system.

**What it does:** Helps you fall asleep faster, stay asleep longer and wake up feeling refreshed instead of feeling like having just lain in bed with your eyes closed for eight hours.

**The reality check:** This isn't some magic sleep potion. If you're still scrolling Instagram with the brightness on full blast while necking espresso at 9 p.m., no amount of magnesium is going to save you. But if you've sorted the basics (light, temperature, caffeine cut-off), then magnesium can be the thing that takes your sleep from average to gold standard.

Your evening routine isn't just about what you avoid, it's about using food and supplements strategically to work with your body's natural wind-down process. Smart carbs help make sleepy hormones. Magnesium helps everything relax.

Simple biology, massive difference.

# THE 'GOOD, BETTER, BEST' MODEL FOR WHEN LIFE EXPLODES

I can almost hear you thinking, 'This all sounds lovely, but what about when my kid's projectile vomiting at 11 p.m.?' or 'Easy for you to say when I've got a work deadline that means I'm up until 2 a.m. finishing a presentation.'

Your life isn't some zen retreat where everything goes to plan. Sometimes life explodes, and a perfect evening routine becomes about as realistic as expecting your teenager to tidy their own room.

## THE 'GOOD ENOUGH' FRAMEWORK THAT WORKS

Perfectionist thinking will destroy any progress you make. Have you ever had one chaotic night and then thought, 'Well, I've blown it'; then spent the next three weeks at bedtime with your phone glued to your face because, 'What's the point?'

Instead of setting yourself up to fail, thanks to impossible standards, let's be realistic. We need to introduce a crucial permission slip for imperfection. We are not aiming for unreachable perfection; we are aiming for consistency. And to do that, we need a flexible framework that works in the real, messy world. This is the 'Good, Better, Best' nightly ritual, and it's saved my sanity countless times.

### *'Good' (the bare minimum – the lifesaver)*

It's past midnight, you're falling into bed after a chaotic evening, and you have zero energy for a ritual. You have one job. Just one.

- Plug your phone in across the room, not next to your bed. That's it. You've still cast one small but powerful vote for a better night's sleep by removing the temptation to scroll.

### 'Better' (the rapid reset – the realistic)

This is your 15-minute emergency routine after a busy night. It's 10:30 p.m. and you're exhausted. The plan is brutally simple and ruthlessly efficient.

- Do a two-minute 'brain dump' (just list the top three things you need to do or remember for tomorrow).
- Put your phone to charge across the room.

### 'Best' (the spa night – the ideal)

This is the full, 60- to 90-minute 'power-down hour' we outlined above. The lights are dimmed, the tech is off, you do your brain dump list, you have a warm bath. You get into bed and read for five minutes. Or simply lie there enjoying the comfort of your bed. This is the goal on a good, calm day. It's the gold standard you aim for when you can.

It's extremely important to rout out the all-or-nothing thinking that holds most people back.

- **Before:** 'I didn't do my full routine so I've failed. Might as well scroll Instagram until 2 a.m.'
- **After:** 'Couldn't do the spa routine, but I did the 15-minute version. That's still a win.'

One chaotic Tuesday doesn't have to derail your entire week. One sick kid doesn't have to ruin all your progress. One work crisis doesn't mean you're back to square one. The reality is that life is messy. Your sleep routine needs to be flexible enough to work with that mess, not against it.

The people who transform their sleep long term aren't the ones with a perfect routine; they're the ones who've mastered being consistently imperfect instead of occasionally perfect.

# THE SLEEP TROUBLESHOOTING GUIDE

You've sorted your evening routine, you're switching off an hour before bed, but your sleep is still a nightmare. Don't panic, there are some specific situations that need their own game plan.

## TWEAK YOUR SLEEP WITH YOUR CYCLE

At certain stages of your menstrual cycle, sleep can feel like a battlefield due to the underlying hormonal chaos. But you can use your cycle as a roadmap, as your insulin sensitivity and sleep architecture naturally change throughout the month. The week before your period (the luteal phase) is often the trickiest. Progesterone is high, which can make you feel more tired, but a drop in serotonin can also disrupt sleep and drive cravings. The luteal phase is the perfect time to be more intentional with your 'sleepy carb' at dinner as the extra carbohydrate support can help boost serotonin, mitigating PMS symptoms and improving your sleep quality when you need it most. Listening to your body and leaning into a slightly higher carb intake in the evenings during this phase is not a failure; it's a smart, hormonally aware strategy.

## SHIFT WORKERS: CREATING YOUR OWN NIGHT

If you work nights, you are essentially living in a permanent state of jet lag. Your internal body clock (circadian rhythm) is in a constant battle with the sun. The key is not to fight it, but to create powerful, consistent 'anchor cues' that signal sleep time to your brain, regardless of what time it is.

- **Master the blackout:** Your bedroom must be a cave. Invest in high-quality blackout curtains. Cover every tiny light from chargers or smoke detectors with electrical tape.

- **Create anchor cues:** Your wind-down routine becomes even more critical. It's your artificial sunset. Do the same things in the same order every 'night' when you get home, even if it's 8 a.m. Maybe it's a warm shower, a specific herbal tea or reading a chapter of a book. These rituals become powerful cues that tell your brain it's time to produce melatonin.
- **Don't flip your schedule on days off:** I know it's tempting to be 'normal' on your non-working days, but this social jet lag will destroy you. Keep your sleep times consistent.

## THE ELEPHANT IN THE BEDROOM: ALCOHOL

Whilst getting to grips with winding down, there's a giant, wine-glass-shaped elephant in the room that we need to address. For millions of women, a glass (or two) of wine in the evening is the go-to tool for stress relief. It feels like it helps you switch off, relax and fall asleep faster. And you're not wrong. Alcohol is a sedative. It can, and often does, help you to fall asleep. But here's the problem: it absolutely destroys the quality of your sleep.

### *What happens*
- Alcohol knocks you out initially (sedative effect).
- It stops you getting into proper deep sleep and REM sleep.
- As your body processes the alcohol during the second half of the night, it releases stress hormones (adrenaline and cortisol) to deal with the blood sugar crash.
- Cue the classic 3 a.m. wake-up where you jolt awake feeling hot, your heart pounding and your mind racing.

I am not telling you to give up alcohol forever, but again, this is about being informed and strategic. Here are the rules for enjoying a drink without completely sabotaging your sleep.

- **The 90-minute rule:** The most important rule is to create a buffer between your last sip of alcohol and your head hitting the pillow. Aim for a minimum of 90 minutes. This gives your liver a head start on metabolising the alcohol, reducing its impact on your sleep.
- **The hydration sandwich:** For every alcoholic drink you have, have a full glass of water. This helps to counteract the dehydrating effects of alcohol, which can further disrupt your sleep.
- **Be a scientist:** Use a sleep tracker app (or just your own perception) as a data tool. Notice the difference in your sleep quality and your next-day energy and cravings on the nights you drink versus the nights you don't.

This isn't about judgment; it's about gathering the data to make empowered choices.

## What to do with your data

- **If you sleep worse and feel terrible the day after drinking:** Consider whether the temporary relaxation given by alcohol is worth the sleep disruption and next-day fatigue. You might decide to limit alcohol to weekends or special occasions.
- **If you notice increased cravings the day after drinking:** This is your blood sugar rollercoaster in action. Plan ahead with protein-rich meals the next day to stabilise your appetite.
- **If you sleep fine using the 90-minute rule:** You've found your sweet spot. Stick to this timing and amount.
- **If even small amounts of alcohol disrupt your sleep:** You might be particularly sensitive to alcohol's effects. Consider alcohol-free alternatives for your evening wind-down routine.

## TROUBLESHOOTING YOUR NIGHT: THE 3 A.M. WAKE-UP PLAN

Waking up in the middle of the night, heart pounding, is infuriatingly common, especially for women with hormone or blood sugar issues. It is often caused by a nocturnal blood-sugar dip. Your body perceives this as an energy crisis and releases cortisol to bring your blood sugar back up, which is what jolts you awake.

### *The fix*

- **Look at your dinner:** Ensure your last meal of the day is balanced, with adequate protein and fat to provide slow-release energy throughout the night.
- **The pre-bed snack (if needed):** For some people, a small snack about an hour before bed can be the solution. It must be the right kind. A small spoonful of almond butter or a handful of nuts provides fat and protein to keep your blood sugar stable overnight.
- **The 'no phone' rule:** When you wake up, the worst thing you can do is look at your phone. The light tells your brain it's morning, and scrolling will just fire up your anxious mind. The rule is: do not touch your phone. Lie in the dark, practise some deep breathing (like the 4-7-8 breath), and speak to yourself kindly, telling yourself everything's okay.

> **THE 4-7-8 BREATH**
>
> Inhale through your nose counting to 4, hold that breath counting to 7, then push all the air out through your mouth, counting to 8. This switches your nervous system from 'alert mode' to 'chill mode' and drops your stress hormones.
>
> Do this three to four times and you'll actually feel your body relax.

You understand that sleep isn't just 'rest time', it's when your brain gets power-washed, your hormones reset and your metabolism decides whether it's going to work with you or against you the next day.

You've got your switch-off hour sorted. You know how to create the perfect sleep cave. You understand why that 3 a.m. wake-up happens and what to do about it. Most importantly, you've learned that good sleep isn't about perfect conditions, it's about working with your specific situation instead of fighting it.

# YOUR THIRD ACTION PLAN: THE 7-NIGHT WIND-DOWN RITUAL

**The mindset shift:** Rest isn't weakness – it's requirements. Your body transforms while you sleep, not while you scroll. You're protecting your progress, not being lazy.

**The goal:** Create your own 'power-down hour' ritual by choosing at least three items each evening from the checklist below. For the next seven nights, your only task is to perform your three choices as a simple, repeatable sequence.

**The task:** Your power-down ritual checklist (choose your 3+ non-negotiables):

- **The light shift:** 90 minutes before bed, dim the main lights and switch on lamps.
- **The tech curfew:** 60 minutes before bed, put your phone on airplane mode and plug it in across the room. No more scrolling in bed.
- **The caffeine curfew:** Set a hard stop for all caffeine at 2 p.m.
- **The brain dump:** 30 minutes before bed, spend five minutes writing down your to-do list and any worries for tomorrow.
- **The warmth signal:** Take a warm bath or shower 60 minutes before bed to help your body temperature drop.
- **The sleepy fuel:** Have your magnesium supplement or a calming, caffeine-free tea (like chamomile or peppermint).

> **The practice:** Track your data.
>
> Each morning, in your notebook, track two simple things (1 = lowest end of the scale (poor) and 10 = best (brilliant)):
>
> - **Sleep quality (1–10):** How well did you sleep?
> - **Morning energy (1–10):** How did you feel when you woke up?
>
> ## HOW TO USE YOUR SCORES:
>
> - **7–10 ratings:** Whatever you did last night, do it again!
> - **4–6 ratings:** One thing needs tweaking – try swapping out one ritual tomorrow.
> - **1–3 ratings:** Your body is telling you 'nope' – change at least two things.
>
> You're not aiming for perfection every single night. You're looking for the patterns that regularly get you to six or above.
>
> By the end of the week, having tried a few different combinations, you'll have proof of what works for your body, instead of just guessing.

Your sleep foundation is now solid. You're not fighting your biology anymore; you're working with it.

Here's what happens next: you take everything you've learned – the hydration timing, the blood sugar balance and now the sleep optimisation – and you let them work together. Because that's when the magic happens: when these systems start supporting each other, instead of you having to perfect each one separately.

# MILESTONE 1: FOUNDATION KNOWLEDGE COMPLETE

Okay, let's have an honest moment of reflection. You're a few chapters in. You've absorbed a lot of information about sleep, hormones, and how your body works. Your brain is probably buzzing with all the things you are, or could be, doing differently.

And, right about now, a little bit of boredom might be creeping in if you are following the suggested systems. The initial excitement might have worn off, and this is where the journey can start to feel like a chore.

This is the perfect time to level up.

What I've learned from working with hundreds of women is that the ones who succeed don't try to change everything at once. They master the knowledge first, then build the habits systematically.

You're still building the foundation. Keep reading. See how everything connects, and when you're happy with it all, we're going to embark on a 4-week challenge. Each week will have a specific focus, and by the end, you'll have built a complete system working in harmony with your body.

But before we dive in, I need you to make me one promise: you're going to treat everything you record during the challenge as *neutral data*, not a report card on whether you're a good or bad person.

If you discover you're eating out of boredom every single evening? That doesn't make you weak or broken. It makes you someone who needs a better evening routine.

If your energy is consistently a 2/10 by the afternoon? That doesn't mean you're lazy or defective. It means your body is crying out for better support.

This challenge isn't about judging yourself. It's about getting curious about how your body works. You're a scientist studying your own biology – be objective, be kind, and remember that every piece of information is just data to help you build a better system.

No shame, no guilt; just genuine curiosity about the amazing machine that is your body.

## WEEK 1: THE DETECTIVE MISSION – GATHERING YOUR DATA

**Your focus this week:** Becoming an expert observer of your own biology.

This isn't about changing everything, it's about understanding your patterns so you can work with them instead of against them.

### MISSION 1: THE MORNING HUNGER AUDIT

Before you eat breakfast, pause for 30 seconds and ask: 'On a scale of 1 to 10, how hungry am I, really?'

- 1 = 'I could take it or leave it.'
- 10 = 'I'm about to eat my own arm.'

Just jot the number down, then eat one of the breakfasts from the breakfast blueprint (page 45).

## MISSION 2: THE AFTERNOON ENERGY CHECK

Between 2 and 4 p.m., pause and ask: 'What's my energy doing right now?' Instead of automatically reaching for coffee or a snack, try a 10-minute walk first. This isn't exercise – it's an experiment to see if you can shift your energy with movement.

## MISSION 3: THE CRAVING DECODE

When a craving hits, pause and ask: 'Is this physical hunger or emotional hunger?'

- **Physical:** 'My stomach is actually rumbling.'
- **Emotional:** 'I'm not hungry, I'm bored/stressed/procrastinating.'

Just identify it – you don't have to fight it or give in.

**End of week 1:** Review your patterns and insights. What did you learn about your body's signals?

### *End of week 1 analysis – what your patterns mean*

- **Consistently low morning hunger (1–4):** You might be eating too late or too much at night. Try stopping food three hours before bed.
- **Always starving in the morning (8–10):** Your blood sugar crashed overnight. Add protein to your evening meal.
- **Afternoon energy consistently low (1–5):** Your lunch isn't sustaining you. Add more protein and fat.
- **Emotional cravings dominate:** Stress is driving your eating. Focus on stress management techniques before tackling food.

## WEEK 2: THE HYDRATION FOUNDATION

**Your focus this week:** Mastering your hydration and energy baseline.

**Your daily target:**

- Start each day with the **morning salt water elixir** before anything else (not just plain water).
- Aim for clear or pale yellow urine by the afternoon.
- Notice how your energy, skin and cravings change.

**Continue from week 1:** Keep doing your morning hunger audits and afternoon energy checks, but now you're building the foundation of proper hydration.

**Track daily:** Morning energy level (1–10) and afternoon energy level (1–10). Watch how hydration affects these numbers.

### What your hydration numbers mean

- **Morning energy improving (6+ vs previous 4–5):** Your hydration protocol is working.
- **Afternoon energy staying low despite hydration:** Look at your lunch composition – you need more protein.
- **No change in energy:** You might need to increase your salt ratio or check your sleep quality.

## WEEK 3: THE BLOOD SUGAR MASTERY

**Your focus this week:** Implementing the craving-control sequence.

**Your daily mission:** Practise the suggested food order at each meal:

1. Fibre (veggies) first.
2. Protein/fat second.
3. Carbs last.
4. Move for 10 minutes after eating (even if it's just tidying up).

**Continue from weeks 1 and 2:** Maintain your hydration habits and body awareness, but now you're actively managing your blood sugar, too.

**Track daily:** Energy levels before, and 2 hours after, each meal. Craving intensity throughout the day (1–10 scale).

### What your meal scores tell you

- **Energy drops 2 hours after eating:** You ate carbs first or didn't have enough protein/fat.
- **Steady energy after meals:** The sequence is working for your body.
- **High cravings (7+ throughout the day):** You're still not eating enough at meals or need to increase protein portions.

## WEEK 4: THE SLEEP OPTIMISATION

**Your focus this week:** Implementing your switch-off hour protocol. Make sure you're continuing with your 3 chosen non-negotiables that you selected on page 74.

**Continue from weeks 1–3:** Maintain all your new protocols while adding sleep optimisation to the mix.

**Track daily:** Sleep quality (1–10) and morning energy (1–10).

### *What your sleep numbers reveal*

- **Sleep quality 7+ but morning energy still low:** Check your room temperature or consider undergoing a sleep study.
- **Sleep quality improving, but slowly,** Keep tweaking your three non-negotiables – try different combinations.
- **No improvement after week 1:** Your main sleep disruptors might be stress or nutrition-related, not routine-related.

Every Sunday, spend 10 minutes reviewing your week:

1. What pattern did you notice?
2. What felt easy this week?
3. What felt challenging?
4. What one thing will you focus on improving next week?

By the end of these four weeks, you won't just have better habits – you'll have developed the most important skill of all: **the ability to listen to your body and respond appropriately.**

You'll know:

- What your body's hunger signals feel like.
- How to use movement to shift your energy.
- How proper hydration affects your entire system.
- How to eat in a way that keeps your blood sugar stable.
- How to create sleep conditions that restore you.

# CHAPTER 4
# THE BALANCE BANK

For years, you will have probably lived under the tyranny of a tiny, judgmental food accountant who lives in your phone. You know the one: every morning, he hands you a strict budget of numbers, and you spend the rest of the day in a state of low-grade anxiety, trying not to 'overspend'. You carefully weigh your chicken breast, you scan the barcode on your yogurt, you meticulously log every single bite. A coffee with a splash of milk? Better log it. Those three almonds you grabbed walking past the kitchen table? Log them too. That single, sad-looking rice cake you had at 4 p.m.? Definitely logging that pathetic excuse for a snack.

For a few days, it would have felt good. Scientific. You felt in control. But then, real life, in all its complex, unpredictable glory, happens. A colleague brings in homemade brownies for your birthday. Your partner cooks a surprise dinner. Your friends suggest a spontaneous trip to the pub.

Suddenly, the system shatters. How many calories are in a homemade brownie? Do you dare ask your partner if he weighed the olive oil? The accountant in your pocket starts sending you passive-aggressive notifications, shaming you for not 'completing your diary'. You're filled with a sense of panic and failure. So, you do what any sane person would do. You fire him. You delete the app, declare the whole thing a miserable failure, and go back to square one, convinced that you are the problem.

Let me be clear – you are not the problem. The system is the problem. Obsessive calorie counting is soul-destroying, unsustainable, and, for the most part, completely unnecessary.

On the other hand, you've also heard wellness gurus breezily claim that 'calories don't matter at all! Just eat clean!' This is also a lie. It's a convenient fantasy that leads to its own special kind of confusion, where you're drinking 'healthy' smoothies packed with 800 calories of fruit and nut butter and wondering why your jeans still don't fit.

The truth, like most things in life, lies in the messy middle. Calories matter, but hormones matter more. The *quantity* of your food has an impact, but the *quality* and *composition* have a far greater one. So, what if we could create a system that respected both? A system that gives you the structure and awareness of tracking, but without the maths, the obsession and the misery? A system that takes two seconds, requires no app, and focuses on the hormonal impact of your food?

Welcome to the balance bank. It's time to fire your food accountant for good.

## THE THREE TIERS OF FOOD: BUILDING A HIGH-SCORING PLATE

To make putting together these nutritious, high-scoring plates easy, we are going to categorise foods into three simple tiers.

Again, this isn't about 'good' vs. 'bad'. It's about understanding the role each food plays.

### TIER 1: FOUNDATION FOODS (YOUR NON-NEGOTIABLES)

These are nutrient-dense, single-ingredient foods that should anchor every meal. Your 'slow logs', packed with protein, fibre, healthy fats, vitamins and minerals.

They provide your protein, fibre and fat points. Here are some examples:

- **Foundation proteins:** Chicken breast, turkey, all types of fish (salmon, cod, tuna, prawns), lean beef, eggs, Greek yogurt, cottage cheese, tofu, edamame.
- **Foundation fibre:** This is an all-you-can-eat buffet of vegetables. Broccoli, spinach, kale, cauliflower, asparagus, peppers, onions, mushrooms, courgettes, beetroot, lettuce, rocket, cucumber. The more colour and variety, the better.
- **Foundation fats:** Avocado, nuts, seeds, olive oil, olives.

## TIER 2: SMART CARBS (STRATEGIC ENERGY)

These are great, healthy, whole foods – the energy-dense sources of carbohydrates. They are the 'paper for the fire', providing essential energy for your brain and workouts. We love them, but we use them strategically.

- **Smart carbs:** Potatoes (all varieties), sweet potatoes, brown/white/wild rice, quinoa, oats, sourdough, beans, lentils, chickpeas and all fruits.
- **Tiny upgrade:** You can make your tier 2 carbs even smarter. When you cook and then cool starchy foods like rice or potatoes, you increase their resistant starch, which is a type of fibre that is brilliant for your gut health and has a gentler impact on your blood sugar. So, a cold potato salad or reheated rice is a tiny but powerful upgrade.

## TIER 3: 'FUN' FOODS (THE JOYFUL EXTRAS)

This is everything else. Pizza, cake, biscuits, chocolate, crisps, pastries, ice cream. Let's be crystal clear: these foods are not 'bad'. They are not 'cheats'. They are a normal and joyful part of a balanced, happy life. The key distinction is their purpose. These foods are for pleasure, not for fuel. They don't offer much in the way of nutrients, and they have a significant impact on your blood sugar. We acknowledge them, we enjoy them and we have a smart strategy coming up for how to handle them.

## INTRODUCING YOUR BALANCE SCORE: THE 5-POINT SYSTEM

The balance bank is not about counting calories. It's about scoring your meals. We are going to give every plate of food a simple balance score from 0 to 5. Your goal is not to stay under a calorie limit, but to deposit high-scoring, hormonally balanced meals into your 'bank' when you eat.

Think of your body like a high-performance car. Calories are the total amount of fuel you put in the tank. The balance score is the *quality* of the fuel. Is it the cheap, dirty petrol that makes the engine sputter and stall, or is it the premium fuel that makes it purr?

A high-scoring meal is premium fuel. It keeps your blood sugar stable, your energy high and your cravings quiet. A low-scoring meal is dirty petrol. It creates hormonal chaos, leaves you feeling tired and hungry, and signals to your body to store fat. We are now going to understand fuel quality by scoring a plate of food. You get one point for each of the following five elements present in your meal:

1. **Protein point:** Is there a significant source of protein? (The anchor.)
2. **Fibre point:** Is there a significant source of fibre from non-starchy vegetables? (The buffer.)

3. **Fat point:** Is there a source of healthy fat? (The satisfier.)
4. **The sequence point:** Did you eat your fibre first? (The hormonal hack.)
5. **The quality point:** Was the meal unprocessed and cooked from scratch? (The foundation point.)

A perfect, gold standard plate scores a 5/5. This is a meal that ticks every single box. A takeaway pizza might score a 0/5 or 1/5. It's not 'bad' – it's just a low-scoring deposit. Our goal? To make more high-scoring deposits than low-scoring ones over the week.

## YOUR CAPSULE SHOPPING LIST

Okay, the tiers make sense on paper, but what does this look like when you're standing in the middle of the supermarket on a Tuesday evening, feeling overwhelmed by the sheer number of options and the beautiful sight of the biscuit aisle?

Let's make this simple. We are going to build your capsule shopping list. This will be a list of the versatile, easy-to-use, all-star items from each tier that will form the backbone of your high-scoring meals.

Let's master the basics first – here are your foundation go-tos.

### TIER 1: PROTEIN, FIBRE AND FAT POWERHOUSES

- **Eggs:** The ultimate fast food. Always have a box to hand.
- **Greek yogurt:** Your go-to for a high-protein breakfast or snack.
- **Chicken breasts or turkey mince:** Your versatile weekday dinner heroes.

- **Frozen salmon fillets or tinned tuna:** For a quick hit of protein and healthy omega-3 fats.
- **Cottage cheese:** High protein, versatile.
- **Tofu or tempeh:** Versatile protein that takes on any flavour.
- **Lentils (dried or tinned):** Quick-cooking protein and a fibre powerhouse.
- **Chickpeas (tinned):** Perfect for salads, curries or roasted snacks.
- **Hemp seeds or pumpkin seeds:** Easy protein boost for any meal.
- **Coconut yogurt (unsweetened):** For those avoiding dairy.
- **Plant-based protein powder:** Quick breakfast or snack option.
- **Nuts and nut butters:** Almonds, cashews, natural peanut butter.
- **Beans (black, kidney, cannellini):** Affordable protein and high in fibre.
- **A big bag of spinach or rocket:** You can wilt this into anything or use it as a base for a salad in seconds.
- **A head of broccoli:** Versatile, nutrient-dense and brilliant roasted.
- **A bag of frozen mixed peppers:** Already chopped. A lifesaver for stir-fries and omelettes.
- **A bottle of extra-virgin olive oil:** For dressings and drizzling.
- **Avocados:** The king of healthy fats.
- **A bag of almonds or walnuts:** For snacking and sprinkling.

## TIER 2: STEADY CARBS

- **A pouch of pre-cooked quinoa or brown rice:** An absolute game-changer for a quick and easy lunch.
- **All sweet potatoes:** More nutrient-dense and gentler on your blood sugar than white ones.
- **A bag of frozen berries:** Perfect for adding to yogurt bowls or protein shakes without a huge sugar hit.
- **A bunch of bananas or a bag of apples:** Your easy, portable carb source.

Your mission for your next food shop is simple: make sure your trolley is at least 70 per cent full of these tier 1 and tier 2 items. If you have these staples in your house, you are never more than 10 minutes away from banking a high-scoring, gold-standard meal.

## TIER 3 FOODS: THE FOUR PS METHOD – HOW TO HANDLE 'FUN' FOODS LIKE AN ADULT

When it comes to tier 3 foods, we don't need restriction, we need a plan. This is the four Ps method: portion, planning, pairing and pace.

1. **Portion:** You can have the cake. But you probably don't need the whole cake. Decide on a sensible portion *before* you start eating. One slice, not three. Same goes for the crisps. A handful of crisps from a bowl, not the whole family-sized bag.
2. **Planning:** The *timing* matters. A piece of chocolate in the afternoon when your willpower is low is dangerous. That same piece of chocolate as a planned dessert after a balanced dinner is a joyful, controlled experience.
3. **Pairing:** Never eat a 'fun' tier 3 food by itself and on an empty stomach. This is like sending a toddler into a china shop unsupervised. Always pair it with a source of protein or fat to reduce the blood sugar spike. Want that biscuit? Have it after a protein-rich meal, not as a standalone 3 p.m. snack.
4. **Pace:** Savour it. Eat it slowly. Put your fork down between bites. Taste it instead of inhaling it. When you eat something mindfully, you are often satisfied with a much smaller amount.

## THE DAILY VS. WEEKEND CHOICE

Okay, so we have a plan for *how* to handle 'fun' tier 3 foods, but the big, nervously asked question remains: how often can I have them?

The old diet culture rules have probably left you with a raging case of food-related anxiety. You're thinking, 'Is it better to have a tiny bit of chocolate every day, or should I save it all up for a big blowout on Saturday night? Which is the "right" way? I don't want to get this wrong!'

There's no single 'right' way. But the most successful women fall into one of two camps.

## 1. THE DAILY CHOICE

This is for the woman who needs a little bit of something fun every day to feel sane, happy and not deprived; the one whose idea of going a whole week without a single taste of chocolate is her personal version of hell. If that's you, then you're in the daily camp. Your strategy is to use the four Ps method on a small portion of high-quality tier 3 food, daily.

### What makes a 'high-quality' fun food?

You probably know most of these already, but seeing them as simple swaps makes it easier to upgrade your choices without completely changing what you eat.

- Dark chocolate (70 per cent+ cocoa) instead of milk chocolate.
- Homemade biscuits instead of mass-produced packaged ones.
- Fresh bakery cake instead of supermarket sponge cake.
- Good-quality ice cream with simple ingredients instead of cheap processed versions.
- Craft beer or decent wine instead of cheap alternatives.
- Proper pizza from an Italian restaurant instead of a basic frozen pizza.

**The simple rule:** Choose the version that has fewer ingredients, tastes better and feels more *special*. If you're going to have a treat, make it worth it.

This isn't about mindlessly grazing on office biscuits; it's an intentional ritual. It's the two delicious squares of dark chocolate you savour after your balanced dinner. It's the single, perfect biscuit you have with your afternoon cup of tea, eaten slowly and with genuine enjoyment.

The key is that the portion is small, the planning is smart (e.g. never on an empty stomach) and the pleasure is high. It's a tiny, daily deposit into your joy bank that keeps your cravings from building up into an unmanageable binge.

## 2. THE WEEKEND CHOICE

This is for the woman who finds it easier to keep things straightforward during the week and prefers to save up her fun for a bigger, more celebratory experience. The thought of a daily treat feels a bit fussy to her; she'd rather have a proper slice of pizza. If that sounds familiar, you're in the weekend camp. Your strategy is to make gold standard, high-scoring deposits into your balance bank from Monday to Friday. Then, on Saturday night, you use the four Ps method to mindfully enjoy a bigger tier 3 meal.

Maybe it's going out for pasta with your partner, or having a couple of slices of takeaway pizza and a glass of wine with friends? The key is that it's planned, intentional and savoured. It's not a guilt-ridden 'cheat meal'; it's a joyful, conscious part of your balanced week. It's the spotlight moment you look forward to, which makes the weekday consistency feel easier and worthwhile.

Neither of these choices is better than the other. They are just different styles. The only 'wrong' thing to do would be to pick the one that doesn't work for you and which leaves you feeling deprived or out of control. Your job is to pick the one that makes you feel powerful, sane and in charge of your own choices.

> **FROM BRONZE TO GOLD: MEAL MAKEOVERS**
>
> Let's see how you could upgrade your food choices in the real world. By making a few simple changes you could deposit more gold standard meals in the bank. If you need to, have a quick refresher of page 83, and then read on.
>
> *Breakfast*
>
> - **Bronze breakfast:** A bowl of cereal with milk. No significant protein, fat or fibre. No sequence. Processed. It's a paper fire that guarantees a mid-morning energy crash. **(Score 0/5)**
> - **Gold standard makeover:** 150g Greek yogurt (Protein point) mixed with 1 tablespoon ground flaxseed (Fibre point), topped with a handful of nuts (Fat point). Eat a spoonful of the flax-yogurt mixture first (Sequence point). Add berries at the end, treating them as your carb component. Made from whole ingredients (Quality point). Rather than eating it in a rush on the go, you sit down with a cup of tea and eat it slowly (Pace). **(Score 5/5)**
>
> *Lunch*
>
> - **Bronze lunch:** A plain pasta salad from a supermarket. (Maybe a Fibre point for a few sad-looking tomatoes. That's it.) The dreaded 3 p.m. slump is inevitable. **(Score 1/5)**
> - **Gold standard makeover:** A large mixed-leaf salad with peppers and cucumber (Fibre point), topped with a grilled chicken breast (Protein point) and an olive oil vinaigrette (Fat point). Eat the salad first (Sequence point). You sit down and make

some actual time to enjoy your lunch, savouring the vegetables and taking note of how you feel (Pace). It's made from scratch (Quality point). You feel light but satisfied, and your energy stays stable all afternoon. **(Score 5/5)**

*Dinner*

- **Bronze dinner:** A large pepperoni pizza. Processed, no sequence, minimal protein/fibre/healthy fat. You scoff it down quickly while watching TV. You feel stuffed, bloated and lethargic. **(Score 0/5)**
- **Gold standard upgrade:** You still want pizza. Great. Let's upgrade it. Before the pizza arrives, you have a big rocket and parmesan side salad with olive oil dressing (eat this first for your Fibre, Fat and Sequence points). You then have two slices of the pizza, which contains a small amount of protein from the cheese and pepperoni (Protein point). You eat the salad slowly first, then take your time with the pizza, chewing properly and putting your fork down between bites (Pace). You've just turned a 0/5 meal into a 4/5 meal, enjoyed the food you craved, and you feel balanced and in control. **(Score 4/5)**

*Common traps and easy wins*

- **The office cake situation:** Someone brings in a cake. The old you either eats it and feels guilty, or resists and feels deprived. The new you applies the four Ps method. You have a small slice (Portion). You have it after your balanced lunch, not on its own (Planning and Pairing). You eat it slowly and enjoy it (Pace). Zero guilt.
- **Kids' parties:** You're surrounded by beige, deep-fried food. The easy win is to eat a high-protein snack *before* you go. This takes the edge off your hunger and makes it much easier to navigate the party food with your sensible brain in charge.

## ESCAPING FOOD JAIL: THE MINDSET SHIFT

We have a system. It's simple. It's logical. It's based on science. But I know what you might be thinking, because I've been there. 'This sounds great, but I've been labelling foods as "good" and "bad" for years. How do I just ... stop? I already know I'm going to feel so much guilt when I eat a bronze meal or a tier 3 food. This just feels like a new way to judge myself.'

If you're feeling this, I want you to know it's completely normal. You have been living in food jail for a long time. The bars of this jail are made of rules, shame and morality. You have been taught that eating a salad makes you a 'good person' and eating a pizza makes you a 'bad person'.

The entire purpose of the balance bank is to tear down that prison.

A 0/5 meal isn't 'bad'. It's simply low-scoring data. Not a reflection of your character or worth as a human being. Just data. Your job is not to be a 'perfect' eater who only ever scores 5/5. That is impossible and, frankly, sounds incredibly boring. Your job is to be a curious scientist. A scientist doesn't get emotional about their data; they simply observe it. They look at their log and say, 'Hmm, interesting. On the days I had a low-scoring lunch, my evening cravings were much higher. That's useful information.'

There *is* no food jail. You are free to eat whatever you want. This system simply gives you the awareness to make choices that will make you feel your best, most of the time. It's about moving from a mindset of restriction and shame to one of awareness and empowerment. When you have a low-scoring meal, you don't punish yourself. You just ask, with kindness, 'What's one small thing I could do to increase the score of my next meal?'

That is the game. And it's a game so straightforward that you just can't lose.

## YOUR NO-NONSENSE FAQs

For the curious ones who want the 'why' behind the 'what', here are the simple answers to your biggest questions.

### 'What's the big deal with cortisol, really?'

Think of cortisol as your body's panicked intern. When you're stressed (from work, bad sleep, over-exercising or under-eating), it runs around pressing the emergency alarm. That alarm tells your body to store fat (especially around your belly) and makes you crave quick, sugary energy to deal with the 'crisis'. Our goal is to keep the intern calm.

### 'Why is protein so important for PCOS and perimenopause?'

Protein is like the responsible adult in the room. For PCOS, it helps stabilise the blood sugar rollercoaster that drives so many symptoms. For perimenopause, as oestrogen declines, our bodies get lazy about holding on to muscle. Eating enough protein is a direct signal to your body to keep that precious, metabolism-boosting muscle.

### 'Do I really need carbs? I thought they were the enemy.'

Carbs are not the enemy; they're a powerful tool that just needs to be used strategically. Think of them as the spark plugs for your engine. You need them for energy, especially for your brain and your workouts. And, as we learned, a small serving of smart carbs at night can be a secret weapon for deep, restorative sleep. It's about the right amount, at the right time.

### 'Which supplements are worth looking into?'

Remember, supplements are the supporting cast, not the star of the show. Your food, sleep and movement are the headliners.

However, a few have solid science behind them. Magnesium glycinate is fantastic for sleep and relaxation. Vitamin D is crucial for almost everything. As always, talk to your doctor before starting anything new.

### 'Why do I feel so ravenous the week before my period?'

It's not your imagination! It's biology. The drop in hormones before your period can cause a dip in your feel-good brain chemical, serotonin. Your brain knows a quick way to get a serotonin hit: carbohydrates. The craving is a real, biological signal from your brain asking for a mood boost. This is why our 'strategic carb' lever works so well (page 53) – it's giving your brain what it's asking for.

# YOUR FOURTH ACTION PLAN: THE 3-DAY BALANCE AUDIT

**The mindset shift:** You're not collecting evidence of failure – you're collecting votes for who you're becoming.

**The goal:** This exercise is not about judgment. It's about building awareness. For the next three days, you are not going to change anything about how you eat. You are simply going to be a detective. After three days, you will have a crystal-clear picture of your current patterns and a dozen simple ideas for how to improve your balance score effortlessly.

**The task:** In your notebook, for every meal and snack you have, you are going to do a quick audit.

- **List the foods:** What did you eat?
- **Assign the tiers:** Label each food as Foundation, Steady Carb or Fun.
- **Give it a score:** Based on the 5-point system, what was your meal's balance score?
- **The upgrade question:** Write one sentence on how you could have easily increased the score. (e.g., 'I could have added a side salad to my pasta,' or 'I could have had some Greek yogurt with my banana.')

You now have a system to build perfectly balanced meals without ever counting a calorie.

You understand the *what*. You've moved from the confusing world of numbers to the empowering world of balance. But one crucial, practical question remains: *How much?*

In the next chapter, I am going to give you the simplest, most straightforward portion control system in the world, using a tool that you already own and take with you everywhere you go.

## CHAPTER 5

# THE HAND-PORTION METHOD

You've done it. You've fired your food accountant. You've embraced the balance bank and you are starting to build beautiful, high-scoring meals. You feel brilliant. You are a strategic, intelligent eater. Then Tuesday night hits. You're standing in your kitchen, staring at a raw chicken breast and a bag of quinoa, and a familiar, anxious thought pops into your head, a ghost from the diet prison you just escaped: 'Okay ... but how much?'

Suddenly, you're having flashbacks to weighing exactly 120g of chicken, measuring one cup of rice, counting out precisely 12 almonds like some sort of kitchen-based mad scientist. You remember the hassle, the obsession, the soul-crushing joylessness of having your dinner dictated by numbers on the kitchen scales.

You know you don't want to go back to that prison, but you're also scared. Those scales felt like a safety net. Without the scales and measuring cups, how do you stop yourself from eating too much? How do you know what a 'portion' is? How can you possibly *trust* yourself to get it right?

This is the final hurdle between you and true food freedom, and we are going to clear it with a tool that is so simple, so elegant and so convenient that you'll wonder how you ever lived without it.

## THE HAND-PORTION METHOD

Forget the kitchen scales, the cups and the spoons. From now on, the only measuring tool you will ever need is the one attached to the end of your own arm.

## WELCOME TO THE HAND-PORTION METHOD*

This is a well-known, scientifically backed, discreet system for controlling your portions anywhere, any time. Your hands are unique to you. They are proportional to your body size, your frame and your energy needs, making them a surprisingly accurate and personalised gauge for your portion sizes. A larger person will have larger hands and thus larger portions; a smaller person will have smaller hands and smaller portions. It's a tailored system you were born with.

Best of all, you take them with you everywhere: to restaurants, to your in-laws' house, on holiday. No one will ever know you're 'measuring' your food. You can finally silence that tiny, judgmental accountant in your head and start eating like a normal, intuitive human being again.

> **WHY THE SCALES WERE HOLDING YOU BACK**
>
> For years, my kitchen scales were both my most trusted friend and my cruellest enemy. That little plastic dictator sat on my kitchen counter, deciding whether I was being 'good' or 'bad' every single day.
>
> The madness of it all still gets me. The anxiety of getting the grams of oats exactly right, tapping tiny flakes off the spoon. The shame of weighing birthday cake when I thought nobody

---

\* Dr Kazzim Mawji came up with this method – calling it the 'Zimbabwe hand jive', to help with portion control.

was looking. The mental gymnastics of trying to calculate the calories in a meal my friend had cooked for me – totally disconnecting me from the joy of the moment.

Those scales promised me precision. They promised me control. What they delivered, though, was obsession. It tied my self-worth to meaningless numbers and systematically destroyed the one thing I desperately needed: trust in my own body and judgment.

Maybe you know this feeling: letting go of your tracking app can feel terrifying, like taking the stabilisers off your bike for the first time. But here's the thing: this fear isn't personal failure. It's conditioning.

Diet culture has been whispering toxic messages in your ear for years: 'You can't be trusted. Your appetite is dangerous. Your instincts are wrong. You need an external control because you're incapable of controlling yourself.'

No wonder you don't trust your own judgment. You've been taught not to.

The hand-portion method is your first step towards reclaiming that trust.

## THE SCIENCE: YOUR INTERNAL MEASURING TOOL

The success of this portioning method lies in its pure simplicity. Traditional calorie counting focuses only on the amount of energy in food, but your body's experience of hunger and fullness is dictated by two key factors: food volume and macronutrient balance.

- **Food volume:** Our digestive system has stretch receptors in both the stomach and intestines that send 'I'm full' signals to the brain when physically stretched. However, satiety also depends on chemical signals from nutrients and hormones. This is why a massive bowl of salad (high volume, low calories) can trigger mechanical fullness signals, while a tiny brownie (low volume, high calories) may satisfy chemical/energy sensors but not provide the same physical fullness sensation.
- **Macronutrient balance:** The right amount of carbohydrates, proteins and fats in your diet trigger powerful satiety hormones. These tell your brain you're satisfied, whereas refined carbs spike insulin and mess with hunger hormones, leaving you wanting more.

The hand-portion method is foolproof because it naturally accounts for *both* of these factors, without any maths involved. It's like having a built-in measuring tool for your meals that automatically calibrates for hormonal balance and fullness.

### MARIA'S STORY

Maria was a 42-year-old teacher who had been held hostage by her kitchen scales for the better part of a decade. She couldn't cook a meal without them. She brought them on holiday with her. She once admitted to me, with a deep sense of shame, that she had taken them in her handbag to a friend's dinner party 'just in case'. She was getting results, but she was miserable. Her life revolved around numbers. She was anxious about eating anywhere but her own home. Her partner was also fed up. 'He just wants to cook for me,' she told me, 'but I can't let him because I don't trust that he'll weigh the pasta correctly. It's ruining our relationship.'

> The thought of giving up her kitchen scales was terrifying for Maria: it felt like jumping out of a plane without a parachute. Our first step was to simply use the hand-portion method to 'check her work'. For one week, she weighed her food as normal, and then compared the portions to the size of her hand. The results were a revelation. Her usual 120g of chicken was almost exactly the size of her palm. Her 40g of uncooked oats was a perfect cupped hand. Her 15g of olive oil was pretty much the length of her thumb. She messaged me midweek: 'This is blowing my mind. My hands have known the right amounts all along.'
>
> That was the turning point for Maria. She realised the scales weren't a safety net; they were a prison. And the key to escape was in her own hands. The following week, she put the scales in a cupboard. A month later, she went out for dinner and, for the first time in years, just ordered her food and enjoyed it, using her built-in measuring tool to guide her choices. She didn't just lose weight; she lost a decade of food-related anxiety.

And while we're on the topic of scales ... you may have noticed a (deliberate) lack of mentioning weighing yourself in this book.

### THE WEIGHING YOURSELF REALITY CHECK

I'm not gonna sugarcoat this – the relationship you have with your bathroom scales probably needs some serious work.

Here's the thing about weighing yourself: it's not actually about the scales at all. It's about how you feel, how you look, how your clothes fit, and how confident you become in your own skin.

That number on the scales? It fluctuates daily based on water retention, hormones, digestion and countless other factors that have nothing to do with your actual progress. Your weight can vary 2 to 4 lbs in a single day just from normal biological processes.

Instead of throwing your scales out of the window (I've been tempted), here's what actually works.

If you choose to weigh yourself:

- Do it daily – same time, same conditions.
- Only look at weekly trends, not daily numbers.
- Remember, your scale measures your relationship with gravity, not your worth.

Better progress tracking:

- Progress photos (even if you hate them, your future-you will thank you).
- How your clothes fit.
- Energy levels throughout the day.
- Strength improvements in the gym.
- How you feel in your own skin.

Below is your new measuring system. Simple, portable, yours forever. Your hands are proportional to your body size. Bigger person = bigger hands = bigger portions. Smaller person = smaller hands = smaller portions. It's a personalised system you were born with.

## YOUR HAND-PORTION METHOD

### Your PALM = PROTEIN portion

- **The visual:** Size and thickness of your open palm – fingers not included.
- **This maps to:** Tier 1 foundation proteins like chicken, fish, beef, tofu. A portion size typically provides 20 to 30g of protein, the sweet spot for stimulating muscle repair and sending powerful fullness signals to your brain.

### Your FIST = FIBRE portion

- **The visual:** Size of your closed fist – aim for two fists per main meal.
- **This maps to:** Tier 1 foundation fibre, for example, broccoli, spinach, peppers or salad. Either raw or cooked and don't hold back, as minimal calories are obtained from maximum volume here.

### Your CUPPED HAND = CARB portion

- **The visual:** What you can hold in your cupped hand.
- **This maps to:** Tier 2 steady carbs like cooked rice, pasta, potatoes or fruit. The quantity is often an eye-opener, but is key to managing your blood sugar level and overall energy intake (without spikes and crashes).

### Your THUMB = FAT portion

- **The visual:** From the tip to the first knuckle of the thumb.
- **This maps to:** Tier 1 foundation fats like oils, butter, nut butters, nuts and seeds. Fats are energy-dense, so this visual guide ensures you get all the hormonal benefits without accidentally overdoing the calories.

> ### *Putting it all together*
>
> Picture your dinner plate. A gold-standard, high-scoring, perfectly portioned meal looks like this:
>
> > 1 palm of salmon
> > 2 fists of roasted asparagus and broccoli
> > 1 cupped hand of quinoa
> > 1 thumb of olive oil used to roast the veg
>
> Perfectly balanced. Perfectly portioned. Zero maths required.

## HAND-PORTION HACKS

The concept is simple, but life is messy. Here are some clever, real-world hacks that will make following the hand-portion method feel effortless, even on your most chaotic days.

### *Hitting your veg target without feeling like a rabbit*

- **The smoothie spinach hack:** This is my number one secret weapon. You can add two fists of fresh spinach to any fruit or protein smoothie, and I promise you will not taste it. It completely disappears, adding a huge hit of fibre and essential vitamins and minerals with zero effort.
- **Bulking agents:** Grated courgette almost disappears when cooked into Bolognese, scrambled eggs or anything, really.
- **Batch roast:** On Sundays, take two big baking trays and fill them with chopped broccoli, peppers, onions and aubergine, cauliflower, carrots, butternut squash, Brussels sprouts, courgettes – whichever vegetables you enjoy. Drizzle with a thumb of olive oil, sprinkle with salt, and roast until tender. Keep this in a container in your fridge. You now have a

ready-to-go source of veggies to add to any lunch or dinner in seconds.

## Protein without the maths

Aim to eat a solid palm of protein at each of your three main meals. This will get you most of the way towards your daily target for muscle repair and satiety.

- **The 'yogurt booster':** A fist-sized pot of Greek yogurt is your secret weapon for an easy protein top-up. As a snack or for dessert, this one addition can easily add another 20g of protein to your day.
- **The 'egg on top':** Don't know how to add protein to your avocado toast or your lunchtime salad? Put a boiled or fried egg on top. It's a simple, fast and effective upgrade.
- **Tuna tin rescue:** Keep tins of tuna in your desk/cupboard. Instant palm of protein for any meal.
- **Cottage cheese comeback:** Sounds boring but mix with berries or use as a base for dips – it's a proper protein powerhouse.
- **Home-roasted chicken batch cook:** Roast a whole chicken on Sunday, strip the meat, portion into containers.
- **Rotisserie chicken cheat:** (Check ingredients and avoid those with added oils and preservatives.) Strip the meat, portion into containers. Easy protein all week.
- **Protein powder stealth mode:** Blend into smoothies; stir into porridge; mix into pancake batter.

## Fat control that still satisfies

Some easy tricks to maintain portion control.

- **The 'nuts in a ramekin' rule:** Nuts are fantastic for you, but it's really easy to go from a sensible 'thumb' to a whole handful (or three). The rule is: never eat nuts directly from the bag. Portion

out your thumb-sized serving into a small bowl or ramekin and then put the bag away.
- **The drizzle-don't-drown dollop:** When dressing a salad, pour your thumb-sized portion of olive oil (about 1 tsp) into a small bowl first, then add your lemon juice or vinegar and whisk it together before pouring it over the salad. This prevents the accidental 'glug' that can turn a healthy salad into a calorie bomb.

## ADJUSTING YOUR PORTIONS: TRAINING DAYS VS REST DAYS

Your body is not a static machine; its energy needs change based on your activity levels. Don't worry, the hand-portion method is easily adaptable.

**On strength-training days:** Your body needs more fuel to perform and recover. On these days, you can slightly increase your 'steady carb' portion. Think of it as upgrading from one cupped hand to two. This extra fuel will top up your muscle glycogen stores, helping you feel strong during your workout and aiding recovery afterwards.

**On rest days or cardio-only days:** Your energy demands are lower. On these days, stick to the standard one cupped hand of carbs per meal. This simple adjustment naturally aligns your energy intake with your energy expenditure – a process known as 'carb cycling', but without any of the complicated maths. And here's the thing – unless you're smashing out hour-long high-intensity interval training (commonly known as HIIT sessions), cardio doesn't actually empty your muscles like lifting does. A 30-minute walk or spin class? Treat it like a rest day. Your body doesn't need extra carbs just because you got a bit sweaty.

## YOUR NO-NONSENSE FAQs

*'My partner's hands are huge! If he uses this method, won't he eat too much food?'*

No! He's a bigger person, so his body likely needs bigger portions. The hand-portion method is beautifully self-scaling. He uses his hands, you use yours. The principles of balance remain the same, but the quantities naturally adjust to the individual.

*'I'm not losing weight, so should I use smaller portions than my hands suggest? I'll just use half a palm of protein.'*

Please, trust me on this: 99 per cent of the time, if progress has stalled, the problem isn't that your portions are too big; it's a lack of consistency or, more often, not enough protein and vegetables. Cutting your protein portion will backfire, leading to more hunger and cravings. Before you consider reducing your portions, you must first ask yourself: 'Have I been truly consistent for three weeks, and am I nailing my palm of protein and two fists of veg at almost every meal?' If in doubt, or in a hurry, just remember the simple 'One palm of protein to two fists of veg' and you're good to go.

*'I'm using my hands to measure my main meals, but I'm still mindlessly snacking on crisps and biscuits in the evening.'*

Your snacks need portion control, too! A snack is a 'mini-plate', and if you're having a carb you should always combine it with a protein or fat to keep your blood sugar stable. Use your hands for this, too. For example, a cupped hand of berries with a fist-sized pot of yogurt; an apple (which counts as a cupped hand) with a thumb of almond butter.

# EATING OUT

This is where the hand-portion method truly becomes a game-changer. You can't take your kitchen scales to a restaurant, but you do always have your hands.

- **The burger joint:** Ditch the bun (or eat only the bottom half): the burger patty is your palm of protein. Ask for a side salad instead of chips. Now you have a balanced, high-scoring meal.
- **The wrap takeaway:** Your carb portion is the wrap itself. Your mission is to load it with a palm of protein (chicken or falafel) and as many fists of salad and vegetables as you can possibly cram in there.
- **The sushi restaurant:** The rice is your carb. Focus on sashimi (just the fish – pure protein) and veggie rolls to up your protein and fibre intake. A good rule of thumb: aim for one fist of edamame or a seaweed salad before you dive into the rice-heavy rolls.
- **The mezze platter:** Your palm of protein is the grilled halloumi or chicken skewers. Your fists of veg are the tabbouleh and salads. Your thumb of fat is the hummus and olive oil. Your cupped hand of carbs is the one or two pieces of pitta bread you use to scoop it all up.

## PLATE-BUILDER TEMPLATES

Here are some simple ideas for constructing a perfectly balanced, hand-portioned plate in any situation.

### *The at-home gold standard plate*
- Protein (1 palm): Grilled salmon fillet.
- Vegetables (2 fists): Green beans and a large side salad.

- Smart carbs (1 cupped hand): Small portion of sweet potato wedges.
- Healthy fats (1 thumb): Olive oil to roast the veg and dress the salad.
- Method: Arrange appealingly – dinner sorted.

### The 5-minute work lunch plate
- Protein (1 palm): Pre-cooked chicken breast or tin of tuna.
- Vegetables (2 fists): Big bag of pre-washed mixed salad leaves.
- Smart carbs (1 cupped hand): Cooked quinoa or a piece of fruit.
- Healthy fats (1 thumb): Small thumb of nuts or a mini pot of hummus.
- Method: Combine in a bowl. Done.

### The 'on-the-go' travel plate (a supermarket sweep)
- Protein (1 palm): Packet of pre-cooked chicken slices or a pot of cottage cheese.
- Vegetables (2 fists): Bag of pre-chopped carrot and cucumber sticks.
- Smart carbs (1 cupped hand): Apple or banana.
- Healthy fats (1 thumb): Small bag of almonds.
- Method: You can build a perfectly balanced meal in any petrol station or supermarket with these components. No excuses.

### Your mix-and-match menu

Okay, you have the basics – the templates. Now, let's make building a simple, nutritious meal at home both foolproof and fun. Think of this as your 'build-a-bowl' menu, just like you'd see at your favourite healthy lunch spot.

Your mission is simple: choose one item from at least three of the five columns opposite to create your perfect meal. This is your ultimate cheat sheet for an optimal meal, every single time.

## THE HAND-PORTION METHOD

| 1. Pick your protein (1 palm) | 2. Load up on fibre (2 fists) | 3. Add your smart carbs (1 cupped hand) | 4. Don't forget healthy fats (1 thumb) | 5. Gut health boosters (optional sprinkle) |
|---|---|---|---|---|
| PRO TIP: Choose the best quality you can afford – organic, grass-fed or free-range when possible. Your body will use high-quality protein more efficiently. | PRO TIP: Vegetables with the ® symbol are tastiest roasted at 200°C/400°F with olive oil and salt, until tender. | PRO TIP: Cook and cool starches like potatoes and rice to increase their gut-friendly resistant starch. | PRO TIP: Prioritise omega-3 fats (marked with an *) for their anti-inflammatory power. | PRO TIP: A tablespoon or two is all you need to support your gut microbiome. |
| POULTRY | LEAFY GREENS | STARCHY and ROOT VEG | OILS and DRESSINGS | FERMENTED FOODS |
| Turkey mince or escalope | Spinach (raw or wilted) | Sweet potato ® | Extra-virgin olive oil | Kimchi |
| Chicken breasts or thighs | Rocket | New potatoes (boiled) ® | Avocado oil | Unsweetened kefir |
| FISH and SEAFOOD | Kale (drizzled with oil) ® | Butternut squash ® | Flaxseed oil* | Miso (in soups / dressings) |
| Salmon fillet* | Lettuce (all types) | Carrots ® | Vinaigrette (oil-based) | Apple cider vinegar |
| Cod, hake, pollock or haddock fillet | | Parsnips ® | | Sauerkraut |
| Tinned tuna in oil/water | CRUCIFEROUS POWERHOUSES | | NUTS and SEEDS | Kombucha |
| Sardines* / mackerel* | Broccoli (cut into florets) ® | GRAINS and LEGUMES | Almonds / walnuts* | |
| Prawns / shrimp | Cauliflower (cut into florets) ® | Quinoa (pre-cooked is great) | Pistachios / Brazil nuts | |
| RED MEAT | Brussels sprouts (halved) ® | Brown or wild rice | Chia seeds* / flaxseeds* | |
| Lamb (chops, minced) | Cabbage (thinly sliced) ® | Lentils (all colours) | Hemp seeds* / pumpkin seeds | |

# THE MINDSET DIET

| 1. Pick your protein (1 palm) | 2. Load up on fibre (2 fists) | 3. Add your smart carbs (1 cupped hand) | 4. Don't forget healthy fats (1 thumb) | 5. Gut health boosters (optional sprinkle) |
|---|---|---|---|---|
| Lean beef mince | COLOURFUL FAVOURITES | Chickpeas | Tahini | |
| Steak (sirloin, flank) | Green beans (topped and tailed) | Black beans / kidney beans | | |
| DAIRY and PLANT-BASED | Peppers (deseeded, sliced) ® | | WHOLE FOODS This section is for minimally processed foods or specify 'homemade versions' where applicable | |
| Lentils / beans | Asparagus (snap off woody ends) ® | FRUITS | Avocado | |
| Cottage cheese | Courgette (sliced) | Berries (all types) | Olives | |
| Eggs (4) | Aubergine (cubed) ® | Apple or pear | Homemade pesto (check for good oils) | |
| Tofu or tempeh (firm) | Mushrooms (sliced) | Banana | Dark chocolate (70 per cent+ cocoa) | |
| Greek yogurt (full-fat) | Onions (sliced) ® | Orange or peach | Brewer's yeast | |
| | Tomatoes (all types) ® | Mango, pineapple, grapes, kiwi, melon, etc. | | |

## HOW TO USE THIS MENU: A REAL-LIFE EXAMPLE

It's a Wednesday night, you're tired and you're staring blankly into the fridge.

- **Pick your protein:** You have some frozen salmon fillets. Perfect. Bake one (1 palm).
- **Load up on veggies:** There's a head of broccoli and a bag of spinach. Chop the broccoli into florets to roast or steam (1 fist) and wilt the spinach (1 fist) at the last minute.
- **Add your smart carbs:** A pouch of pre-cooked quinoa is at the back of the cupboard. Easiest decision ever. Heat some up (1 cupped hand).
- **Don't forget healthy fats:** Use olive oil to roast the broccoli or drizzle it on the salmon (1 thumb).
- **Gut health booster (optional):** Add a tablespoon of kimchi on the side for some spicy, gut-friendly goodness.

**The result:** A delicious, perfectly balanced meal of baked salmon, roasted broccoli, wilted spinach and quinoa, topped with a little kimchi. It took you less than 60 seconds to plan, it uses simple ingredients, and it will keep you full, energised and hormonally balanced all evening.

This is the end of not knowing what to make for dinner. You now have a system and a mix-and-match menu that makes healthy eating simple, creative and delicious.

# YOUR FIFTH ACTION PLAN: 7-DAY 'TALK TO THE HAND' CHALLENGE

**The mindset shift:** At your next meal, before you eat anything else, look at the protein on your plate. Hold up your palm next to it. Is your chicken breast, fish fillet or tofu roughly the size of your palm? If not, adjust it. Your palm is your built-in measuring tool for the most important part of your meal.

## DAYS 1–3: THE AUDIT

Knowledge is potential power. Action is *real* power. For one full week, you are going to become a master of this method. This is an observation exercise to build up your intuitive portioning skills.

**The goal:** Getting comfortable and confident with using the hand-portion system.

**The task:** For the next three days, plate your food as you normally would.

**The practice:** Before you take a single bite, stop. Hold your hand up next to your plate. Visually assess each component against the hand-portion guide.

Just notice:

- 'I only had half a fist of vegetables.'
- 'My protein portion is actually bigger than my palm.'
- 'I forgot to add any healthy fats.'
- 'My carb portion could feed three people.'
- 'I'm eating mostly carbs and very little protein.'

Remember: this isn't about being perfect – it's about building awareness of your current patterns so you know what to adjust.

## DAYS 4–7: THE PRACTICE

**The goal:** To experience how a correctly portioned meal *feels*. Notice your energy levels two hours later. Notice your cravings (or lack of) in the evening.

**The task:** For the next four days, actively try to build your plates using the hand-portion method as your guide.

**The practice:** Start with just one meal a day. Look at your hand, and serve your protein, fibre, carbs and fat accordingly.

This audit will be a game changer. You'll notice where you've been over-serving (usually carbs and fats) and under-serving (usually vegetables and protein). This awareness is the foundation of effortless, intuitive eating.

You now have a complete nutrition system that's flexible, travels everywhere and requires zero maths. You know what balanced meals look like and how much to eat.

But good planning will be made much more difficult if your kitchen's a war zone and your cupboards are empty. To make this system automatic and easy, we need your environment working for you, not against you. In the next chapter, we're making your food life completely frictionless with smart shopping and 10-minute meal prep that works.

## CHAPTER 6

# SHOPPING, BATCHING AND 10-MINUTE PLATES

It's 4 p.m. on Sunday. You're standing in the fluorescent nightmare of a crowded supermarket, staring at a wall of yogurts and feeling a familiar sense of dread. Your trolley is half-full of the same old 'healthy' things you buy every week. You have the best intentions. You've bought a forest of broccoli and a mountain of spinach, picturing the vibrant, energetic woman you'll be this week, whipping up nutritious meals from scratch.

But a quieter, more honest voice in your head is already telling you the truth. It knows that by Thursday, that spinach will have transformed into a bag of green, slimy sludge at the back of your fridge. It knows that on Wednesday night, when you get home late and exhausted, the thought of washing, chopping and cooking that broccoli will feel as appealing as assembling flat-pack furniture.

This weekly pattern – optimistic shop followed by the slow decay of good intentions – isn't just frustrating; it's expensive, wasteful and it chips away at your self-belief. Each bag of wilted salad is more evidence for the story you tell yourself: 'I can't stick to it. I'm not organised enough. I don't have time.'

Your problem isn't lack of time or willpower. Your problem is decision fatigue.

Decision fatigue is a real thing. Your brain can only make so many good decisions before it gives up. You are the chief logistics officer (CLO) of your life – you spend your entire day making decisions for your work, your family, your finances. By 5 p.m., your decision-making fuel tank is empty. When you ask your exhausted brain, 'What should I make for healthy dinner tonight?' it does what any overwhelmed brain would do: chooses the easiest option. In our world, easiest is almost always the least healthy – takeaway menu, beans on toast, whatever requires zero thought.

This chapter is about front-loading your success by learning to make all your smart food decisions once a week when your brain is fresh. We're creating a system that makes healthy eating the path of least resistance.

Imagine, one hour on Sunday could save you countless hours of stress during the week. We're going to build your own personal, healthy 'grab-and-go' service, right inside your fridge.

## THE 'RESTAURANT IN YOUR FRIDGE' PHILOSOPHY

When you think of 'food prep', most people think of miserable Sunday afternoons spent portioning out identical, boring meals of dry chicken, limp broccoli and plain rice into a depressing stack of plastic containers.

Think again. That is a food prison, and we are not living that life. Our approach is different. I call it the 'restaurant in your fridge'.

Think about your favourite healthy lunch spot. You walk in, and you see a beautiful array of pre-prepped ingredients behind the counter: grilled meats, roasted sweet potatoes, quinoa, chopped vegetables, delicious sauces. You don't have to cook anything; you just have to make choices. You point and say, 'I'll have a bit of that, a scoop of that, and a drizzle of that, please.' Five minutes later, you have a perfect, delicious, balanced meal.

And that is what we are going to create in your own fridge. We are not prepping full meals. We are prepping *components*. This is the key. By spending one hour every Sunday prepping a few core bases, you give yourself the ultimate gift for the week ahead: the freedom of choice without the burden of cooking from scratch.

## STEP 1: THE STRATEGIC SHOP

It all starts at the supermarket. A chaotic food shop leads to a chaotic week. A planned one sets you up for success. This is your 'capsule wardrobe' shopping list. It's designed to be simple, versatile and to give you everything you need for a week of high-scoring, balanced meals.

Rather than giving you a rigid list, here's how to shop strategically using your build-a-bowl table from page 110:

### *From your protein options (choose 3–4 for the week)*
- Pick what your family actually eats.
- Consider what recipe cards you want to try this week (see pages 124 and 307).
- Ensure variety across the week.

### *From your fibre options (the more the merrier)*
- Choose vegetables you'll actually use.
- Mix fresh, frozen and shelf-stable options.
- Think about prep time available.
- From your smart carbs (choose 2–3).

- Focus on versatile options that work across multiple meals.
- Consider batch-cooking opportunities.

### *From your healthy fats (your staples)*
- Quality extra-virgin olive oil (look for dark glass bottles to protect from light).
- Avocados.
- A bag of almonds or walnuts.
- Any others from your build-a-bowl selection.

### *From your flavour heroes (the game-changers)*
- Good-quality pesto (check ingredients – look for versions made from extra-virgin olive oil, not seed oils).
- Fresh herbs (basil, mint, coriander) and dried spices (turmeric, cinnamon, paprika).
- Low-sodium chicken or vegetable stock.

This connects directly to your recipe cards (see pages 124 and 307) and allows you to customise based on what you actually want to eat this week.

## STEP 2: THE SUNDAY POWER HOUR

This is your appointment with your future self. Put on a great podcast, pour yourself a cup of tea, and get it done. This one hour will buy you back at least five hours of stress during the week.

Your mission is to prep four bases to provide your protein, carbs, vegetables and flavourings for the coming week.

### *Base Prep 1: the protein hub*
10–15 minutes prep time; 15–25 minutes cooking time

**The how:** Take your pack of selected meat or fish. Drizzle with olive oil, sprinkle generously with salt, pepper and any other spices you like. (Paprika, garlic powder and oregano is a great all-purpose mix you can also prepare and store in a jar.) Lay them on a baking tray lined with baking paper. Put them in a preheated oven at 200°C/400°F for about 15 to 25 minutes (cooking times will vary according to size, but thicker cuts may need 25 to 30 minutes), until cooked through. Let them cool, then store whole in a container in the fridge.

**The result:** You now have a ready-to-go, versatile protein source for the next 3 to 4 days.

### *Base Prep 2: the smart carb staple*
5 minutes prep time; approx. 15–20 minutes cooking time
**The how:** While the meat or fish is cooking, choose your carb.

- **Quinoa/rice:** Rinse, put in a pan with double the amount of water, bring to a boil, then simmer until the water is absorbed and they're cooked to your taste. Fluff with a fork and let it cool.
- **Sweet potatoes:** Pierce them a few times with a fork and bake whole alongside the chicken. Or, chop them into wedges, toss with a little oil and salt, and roast them for 15 to 20 minutes.

**The result:** A ready-to-use, blood-sugar-balancing carbohydrate source.

## BASIC CARB PREPARATION METHODS

Note: Serving sizes are based on the hand-portion method – one cupped handful of uncooked grains typically serves one person as a side, or use two cupped handfuls for a main dish base.

### QUINOA (serves 4–6)

- **Amount:** 1 cupped handful of quinoa to 2 cups water.
- **Method:** Rinse quinoa first, bring water to boil, add quinoa, reduce to simmer.
- **Time:** 15 minutes (until water absorbed).
- **Cooked when:** Grains look fluffy and you can see the little 'tails'.

### BROWN RICE (serves 4–6)

- **Amount:** 1 cupped handful of rice to 2 cups water.
- **Method:** Rinse rice until water is clear, bring water to boil, reduce to simmer.
- **Time:** 20–25 minutes (until water absorbed).
- **Cooked when:** Grains are tender, not crunchy.

### SWEET POTATOES

**Whole Baked:**

- **Method:** Pierce with fork 4 or 5 times, bake at 200°C/400°F.
- **Time:** 25–35 minutes (depending on size).
- **Cooked when:** Soft when squeezed gently.

**Chopped Wedges:**

- **Method:** Cut into 2cm wedges, toss with oil and salt.
- **Time:** 15–20 minutes at 200°C/400°F.

- **Cooked when:** Golden and tender when pierced with fork.

**NEW POTATOES**
- **Method:** Halve if large, boil in salted water, or steam.
- **Time:** 12–15 minutes.
- **Cooked when:** Easily pierced with knife.
- **Pro Tip:** All cooked carbs will keep in the fridge for 3 to 4 days.

## *Base Prep 3: The veggie vault*
15 minutes

**The how:** While everything is cooking, chop up the roasting vegetables you've chosen for this week. Toss them with a little oil and salt. When the meat or fish are cooked, put the tray of vegetables into the hot oven and roast for 20 to 30 minutes or until tender and slightly caramelised.

**The result:** A delicious, fibre-rich, ready-to-eat vegetable component.

## *Base Prep 4: Flavour foundations*
5 minutes prep time; keeps for 1 week

These flavour bases transform basic proteins and carbs into meals you'll look forward to. Having these ready means the difference between bland, boring food and something that keeps your tastebuds happy. Make one or two on your prep day and you're sorted for the week.

**Dressing**
- 1 tbsp olive oil + 1 tbsp lemon juice + pinch of salt.

**Pesto sauce**
- Shop-bought: 1 to 2 tablespoons per serving. Look for versions with olive oil as the first fat, not sunflower oil. Check the ingredient list as fewer ingredients = better quality.
- Homemade: Blend 2 cups basil, ½ cup olive oil, ¼ cup pine nuts, 2 garlic cloves and ¼ cup parmesan.

**Hummus and lemon**
- 2 to 3 tablespoons hummus plus a squeeze of fresh lemon juice.

**Soy and ginger sauce**
- 2 tablespoons soy sauce/tamari, 1 teaspoon of fresh grated ginger (or ½ tsp ground ginger).

You now have your own restaurant-style prep in your fridge. The hard work is done. Well done!

## STEP 3: THE 9-MEALS-IN-10-MINUTES WONDER

This is where the magic happens. With your prepped bases, you can now assemble a huge variety of meals in minutes. The hard work is done. Well done!

With your prepped bases, you can now assemble a huge variety of meals in minutes. Mix and match your prepared proteins, carbs, vegetables and sauces to create different combinations throughout the week. The beauty of this system is flexibility – use what you have, combine flavours differently each day, and never get bored.

In your kitchen prep, you can be more precise with measurements than the hand-portion method. Use standard measuring cups for cooking prep, then serve using your hand portions when plating up meals.

The following recipe cards have been created to show just how versatile the system can be – you don't need to be eating the same soggy tuna salad day in day out to see results. I've used chicken as an example, but they'll work with all sorts of protein. Prep a nice batch of protein ahead of time, and mix and match your pairings.

*Recipe card 1: chicken power bowl*

**Prep time:** 5 minutes

1. Place 1 cupped hand of quinoa in a bowl.
2. Top with 1 palm portion of sliced chicken.
3. Add 1 fist of roasted vegetables.
4. Make dressing: 1 tbsp olive oil + 1 tbsp lemon juice + pinch of salt.
5. Add a large handful of fresh spinach.
6. Drizzle dressing over everything.
7. Sprinkle with 1 tbsp pine nuts or almonds.

**Why this works:** Complete protein + complex carbs + healthy fats + fibre + antioxidants

*Recipe card 2: chicken and veggie stir-fry*

**Prep time:** 10 minutes

1. Heat 1 tsp olive oil in a pan.
2. Add 1 palm portion of pre-cooked chicken (cook through for 2 minutes).
3. Add 1 fist of roasted vegetables (warm for 2 minutes).
4. Make sauce: 2 tbsp soy sauce + 1 tsp fresh grated ginger.
5. Pour sauce over chicken and vegetables.
6. Serve over 1 cupped hand of quinoa.
7. Top with a handful of fresh spinach and 1 tbsp chopped almonds.

**Why this works:** Anti-inflammatory ginger + complete amino acids + sustained energy

*Recipe card 3: pesto chicken quinoa salad*

**Prep time:** 5 minutes

1. Let pre-cooked quinoa come to room temperature.
2. Mix 1 cupped hand quinoa with 2 tbsp good-quality pesto.
3. Add 1 palm portion of diced chicken.
4. Mix in 1 fist of roasted vegetables (chopped smaller).
5. Add large handful of rocket or spinach.
6. Drizzle with 1 tsp extra olive oil.
7. Top with 1 tbsp walnuts and cherry tomatoes.

**Why this works:** Brain-healthy omega-3s + sustained energy + gut-friendly fibre

*Recipe card 4: chicken and hummus wrap*

**Prep time:** 5 minutes

1. Take 1 large wholemeal tortilla.
2. Spread 3 tbsp hummus across the wrap.
3. Add 1 palm portion of sliced chicken.
4. Add 1 fist of roasted vegetables.
5. Add handful of fresh spinach or lettuce.
6. Squeeze fresh lemon juice over filling.
7. Drizzle with 1 tsp olive oil.
8. Roll tightly and slice in half.

**Why this works:** Portable + protein + fibre + healthy fats + blood sugar balance

*Recipe card 5: warming chicken and vegetable quinoa bowl*

**Prep time:** 10 minutes

1. Heat 1 tsp olive oil in a pan.

2. Add 1 cupped hand quinoa with 2 tbsp water (warm for 2 minutes).
3. Add 1 palm portion chicken and 1 fist vegetables (properly reheated).
4. Season with salt, pepper and 1 tsp turmeric.
5. Transfer to bowl and add handful of fresh spinach (will wilt).
6. Drizzle with 1 tbsp olive oil mixed with lemon juice.
7. Top with 1 tbsp pumpkin seeds.

**Why this works:** Anti-inflammatory turmeric + warming + hormone-supporting healthy fats

### *Recipe card 6: Greek-style chicken salad*

**Prep time:** 5 minutes

1. Create salad base with large handful of spinach and rocket.
2. Add 1 cupped hand of quinoa.
3. Top with 1 palm portion of chicken.
4. Add 1 fist of roasted vegetables.
5. Make Greek dressing: 1 tbsp olive oil + 1 tsp red wine vinegar + pinch oregano.
6. Add 5 to 6 olives and 1 tbsp crumbled feta cheese.
7. Drizzle dressing over everything.

**Why this works:** Mediterranean diet benefits + probiotics from cheese + antioxidant-rich olives

### *Recipe card 7: protein-packed quinoa 'fried rice'*

**Prep time:** 10 minutes

1. Heat 1 tsp olive oil in a large pan.
2. Add 1 cupped hand quinoa (fry for 2 minutes until slightly crispy).
3. Push quinoa to one side, scramble 1 egg in the empty space.
4. Mix egg through quinoa.
5. Add 1 palm portion diced chicken and 1 fist vegetables.

SHOPPING, BATCHING AND 10-MINUTE PLATES

6. Season with 2 tbsp soy sauce + 1 tsp sesame oil.
7. Top with handful of fresh spinach and 1 tbsp sesame seeds.

**Why this works:** Extra protein from egg + satisfying texture + B vitamins for energy

### *Recipe card 8: Mediterranean stuffed sweet potato*

**Prep Time:** 5 minutes (if you have pre-baked sweet potato)

1. Take 1 medium baked sweet potato, slice open.
2. Fluff flesh with a fork.
3. Top with 1 palm portion of warm chicken.
4. Add 1 fist of roasted vegetables.
5. Make tahini dressing: 1 tbsp tahini + 1 tsp lemon juice + 1 tsp water.
6. Add handful of fresh spinach.
7. Drizzle with tahini dressing.
8. Sprinkle with 1 tbsp chopped almonds.

**Why this works:** Beta-carotene + complete protein + healthy fats + satisfying comfort food feel

### *Recipe card 9: chicken and quinoa soup*

**Prep time:** 10 minutes

1. Heat 1 tsp olive oil in a saucepan.
2. Add 2 cups low-sodium chicken or vegetable stock.
3. Bring to simmer, add 1 cupped hand quinoa.
4. Add 1 fist of roasted vegetables (chopped smaller).
5. Add 1 palm portion of shredded chicken.
6. Simmer for 5 minutes until heated through.
7. Stir in large handful of fresh spinach (will wilt).
8. Finish with 1 tbsp olive oil and fresh herbs.

**Why this works:** Hydrating + warming + easily digestible + nutrient-dense

## PRO TIPS FOR ALL RECIPES

- **Make it fresh:** Add something raw (spinach, herbs, lemon) to every meal.
- **Healthy fat is essential:** Don't skip the olive oil – it helps you absorb nutrients.
- **Customise freely:** Swap vegetables, nuts or seasonings based on what you have.
- **Batch-prep friendly:** All these recipes work well made in larger portions.

You just created nine different meal ideas.

## THE FLAVOUR MATRIX: YOUR SECRET WEAPON AGAINST BOREDOM

'Okay,' I imagine you thinking. 'This is clever. But am I just supposed to eat plain chicken, veg and quinoa with a bit of pesto for the whole week? I'll be bored out of my mind by Wednesday.'

This is a valid concern. The batch-cooking emphasis for the 'restaurant in your fridge' suggestion is only appealing if the food is delicious. The secret to avoiding flavour fatigue is to prep different meals, not by seasoning them with neutral flavours (e.g. salt, pepper and olive oil), but to use a 'flavour hero' to transform your batch cooking into a different meal each night.

As we saw above, your sauces, spices and 'toppers' are your best friends. Here are three simple flavour profiles you can create in seconds to keep things interesting.

| Flavour Profile | Apply to Your Protein | Apply to Your Veggies | Apply to Your Carbs | The Finished Dish |
|---|---|---|---|---|
| Italian-inspired | Reheat the chicken with a spoonful of pesto or tomato passata. | Drizzle with balsamic vinegar for a glaze. Top with a sprinkle of parmesan. | Mix quinoa with fresh basil and cherry tomatoes. | A vibrant Italian-style power bowl. |
| Mexican-inspired | Shred the chicken and mix with a sprinkle of fajita seasoning and a squeeze of lime. | Top with a spoonful of tomato salsa and a slice of avocado. | Mix quinoa with some black beans and sweetcorn. | A deconstructed burrito bowl. |
| Asian-inspired | Drizzle the chicken with a little soy sauce (or tamari) and sesame oil. | Top veggies with a sprinkle of toasted sesame seeds. | Drizzle quinoa with a little soy sauce and top with spring onions. | A delicious, nutrient-packed stir-fry bowl. |

You haven't cooked anything new. You have simply assembled the same three bases in a slightly different way, using a different flavour hero. This is how you eat from the same prep batch all week without ever feeling like you're eating the same meal twice.

## ONE BASE, TWO PLATES

'This is all lovely for me,' you might be thinking, 'but I have a partner and two kids who are not going to eat a quinoa bowl with soy-glazed vegetables. They want spaghetti Bolognese. Am I supposed to make two completely different meals every single night?'

Absolutely not. That is a one-way ticket to burnout. The solution is the 'bridge meal' – that is, cooking *one* core meal and then serving it in two different ways, thereby building a 'bridge' between your family's meal and your own balanced plate. Let's take spaghetti Bolognese as an example.

**Cook one base:** You make a big, delicious batch of Bolognese sauce. To make it a gold standard base, you pack it with extra veggies – grate a carrot and a courgette into the mince, plus add finely chopped mushrooms, celery and peppers. Once cooked down, no one will notice them.

**Serve two ways**
1. **For your family:** You serve their portion of the Bolognese sauce over regular spaghetti. You put a bowl of grated cheese on the table. They are happy.
2. **For you:** Build your own high-scoring plate. Chuck a big handful of spinach on your plate (that's your first fist of veg). Spiralise some courgette into 'courgetti' or just use a veggie peeler to make ribbons. Warm them up in a pan or microwave until they're just soft (avoid turning them into mush!). Need more veg? Add another fist-sized portion (cooked veg shrinks down so you might need it). Then pile on a palm-sized portion of Bolognese sauce for your protein hit, and finish with a thumb-sized sprinkle of parmesan or a drizzle of olive oil for your fats.

**Some more options**
- **Fajita night:** You cook the chicken and pepper filling for everyone. Your family have theirs in flour tortillas with sour cream, tomato salsa and guacamole. You have yours over a bed of salad leaves with the salsa and guacamole, too.
- **Roast dinner:** Everyone has the roast chicken and roasted potatoes, broccoli and carrots. They have theirs with gravy and Yorkshire puddings. You swap the Yorkshires for an extra two fists of the veg.

Job done. Proper balanced plate that'll actually keep you satisfied. And you can apply this strategy to almost anything.

## THE STORAGE MASTERCLASS

'Won't the prepped food get gross and soggy by Wednesday?' This is a valid and crucial question. The success of the restaurant-in-your-fridge concept depends on the food staying appealing to eat. Here are some pro tips for keeping your components fresh.

- **Store components separately:** This is the golden rule. Do not mix everything together into pre-made meals. Keep your cooked protein, your roasted veg, your quinoa and your sauces in separate containers. Assemble your bowl right before you eat. This keeps everything crisp and fresh.
- **Glass is class:** If you can, invest in a set of glass food storage containers. Unlike plastic, they don't stain or absorb odours, and your food will taste fresher.
- **The paper towel trick for greens:** To keep your big bag of spinach or rocket from turning into a slimy mess, open the bag, place a folded piece of paper towel inside, and then seal the bag back up with a clip. The paper towel absorbs the excess moisture that causes wilting. You'll get an extra 3 to 4 days of freshness from your greens.
- **Don't dress your salads:** If you're prepping a lunchbox salad, put your olive oil or dressing in a separate container. Only add it at the last second just before you eat to avoid a soggy, sad desk lunch.

# THE 'I'M KNACKERED' DEFAULTS: YOUR 2-MINUTE EMERGENCY MEALS

Some weeks, a full Sunday 'power hour' is just not going to happen. In this case, aim for a 20-minute emergency prep. The two things to prioritise are a protein source (bake some chicken or hard-boil some eggs) and a washed salad base. If you just have these ready, you can always build a meal.

Some nights, even assembling a bowl feels like too much work. For these moments of extreme fatigue, you need a 'no-cook' emergency default. These are meals you can assemble in under two minutes that are still way better than a takeaway.

### *The rotisserie chicken miracle*

A pre-cooked rotisserie chicken from the supermarket is your best friend.

- A palm-sized portion of chicken.
- A handful of pre-washed salad leaves.
- A drizzle of olive oil.
- Half a tin of black beans (drained and rinsed) or a slice of good bread.

### *The tuna and avocado bowl*

- A tin of tuna + half an avocado, mashed together with a fork.
- A squeeze of lemon.
- A sprinkle of salt.
- Slice of good bread or handful of crackers (carbs).
- Handful of cherry tomatoes.

### *The quick quinoa bowl*

- A handful of ready-to-eat quinoa (from pouch).

- Pot of full-fat cottage cheese.
- Handful of cherry tomatoes.
- Drizzle of olive oil + pinch of salt and pepper.

### *The smoked salmon bagel*
- 1 wholegrain bagel (toasted).
- Cream cheese spread.
- Pre-sliced smoked salmon.
- Handful of rocket leaves.

## THE LIFELINE: YOUR 10-MINUTE SUPERMARKET SWEEP

Let's be realistic. There will be a Sunday when your power hour of prep gets completely derailed. You might have a family emergency, or you might just be so exhausted from a fun weekend that the thought of strategic batch-cooking is laughable.

You wake up on Monday morning with a familiar sense of dread. Your fridge is empty. Your week feels doomed before it's even begun. The old you would have declared the week a write-off and resigned yourself to five days of expensive, unsatisfying and unhealthy takeaway lunches. But you are now the chief logistics officer of your own well-being, and a CLO knows how to pivot brilliantly when the plan goes awry. This is not a crisis. This is a simple logistical problem, and we have an easy solution.

Welcome to the 10-minute supermarket sweep. This is your 'no-cook' emergency prep plan that you can execute on your Monday lunch break or on your way home from work.

Your mission is to go into any major supermarket and be out in under 10 minutes with the components for a balanced, healthy 'restaurant in your fridge' for the next 48 hours.

## THE SUPERMARKET SWEEP

- **Go directly to the protein aisle.** Do not pass Go, do not browse the biscuit aisle. Your first stop is for ready-to-eat protein. Pre-cooked options (turkey, ham, chicken strips, salmon), smoked fish, cottage cheese/Greek yogurt, or tinned beans/lentils for plant-based eaters. Choose what works for you and grab one.
- **Proceed to the fresh produce aisle.** Your target here is zero-effort vegetables. Grab a big bag of pre-washed mixed salad leaves (like spinach or rocket). Then, pick up a bag or pot of pre-chopped 'snacking' veg (like cherry tomatoes, baby cucumbers or carrot sticks).
- **Advance to the grocery aisle.** We need a smart carb source that requires no cooking. Your hero here is a pouch of pre-cooked quinoa, lentils or mixed grains. A tin of chickpeas (drained and rinsed) also works perfectly.
- **Finish with the condiment aisle.** The final part is flavour. Grab a tub of hummus or a bottle of good-quality vinaigrette.

That's it. In less than 10 minutes, you have just created your own deconstructed 'restaurant in your fridge'. You have your protein, your two fists of veg, your cupped hand of carbs and your thumb of fat/flavour. You have everything you need to assemble a perfect, high-scoring lunch and dinner for the next two days.

You haven't failed. You've adapted. You've proven that you can find a solution even when you're starting on the back foot. This is not about being a perfect prepper; it's about being a resourceful problem-solver. And that is a skill that will serve you for life.

# YOUR SIXTH ACTION PLAN: PLANNING FOR A STRESS-FREE WEEK AHEAD

**The mindset shift:** Protecting your energy isn't selfish – it's essential. You can't pour from an empty cup, and saying no to some things means saying yes to yourself.

**The goal:** Your mission is to enjoy the feeling of being organised for the upcoming week by planning, shopping and batching at the weekend. You know your future self will thank you for it.

**The task:** The strategic shop – take the shopping list. Get in, get the goods, get out. No aimless wandering. Operation complete.

**The practice:** Power hour – schedule one hour this Sunday for food prep. Put in your diary a non-negotiable appointment with yourself. If you follow the system and prep three bases (protein, carb and vegetables), you'll be all set for when life gets busy. Put on some music or a podcast, make it enjoyable and know that the batching you do during that one hour will make healthy eating the easiest choice during the week. No more Sunday-night anxiety about an empty fridge. No more Wednesday evening desperation. No more expensive takeaway guilt.

Congratulations. You've built your own personal restaurant in your fridge. Time to enjoy the convenience you just created for yourself – with none of the stress.

# CHAPTER 7

# FUN FOODS WITHOUT THE NEGATIVE SPIRAL

You're doing it. You're drinking your salted water, you're eating your veggies first, you're sleeping more deeply and you're prepping your 'restaurant in your fridge' on Sundays. You're feeling good. You're feeling powerful. You are, for the first time in a long time, feeling in control.

And then it happens. It's your best friend's birthday. Someone places a huge, glorious chocolate cake on the table, and a slice is passed to you. And in that moment, your brain short-circuits. Two competing voices start screaming in your head:

**Voice 1:** 'Don't you dare! Don't you dare touch that cake! You've been so good. This is a trap. This is how it all unravels. One bite and you'll undo all your hard work. Just say no.'

**Voice 2:** 'Go on. You deserve it. You've been so restrictive. What's the point of all this if you can't even have a piece of cake? Just eat it. You can start again on Monday.'

This is the internal battle that has defined every diet you've ever tried. It's a miserable choice between deprivation and guilt: you either resist the cake and feel bitter and resentful, or you eat the cake and feel weak-willed and ashamed. Either way, you lose.

What if there was a third way? A way to eat the damn cake, enjoy every single bite of it, and wake up the next morning feeling zero guilt, zero bloating and completely in control?

Welcome to the final piece of your food freedom puzzle. This chapter is about dismantling the biggest lie diet culture ever told you: the lie that pleasure is the enemy of progress.

The truth is that pleasure is not just a part of the plan; it is the secret ingredient that makes the actions recommended in this book sustainable for life.

So let's give you a simple, powerful, four-step strategy for handling any 'fun food' (those from tier 3, on page 84) – like a slice of cake or a bag of crisps – with the cool, calm confidence of a woman who is truly in charge.

This is how you escape the all-or-nothing spiral for good.

## THE SCIENCE: WHY DEPRIVATION IS A LOSING STRATEGY

For years, you've been taught that the key to success is restriction; to white-knuckle your way through temptation. But this strategy is doomed to fail, for a simple psychological reason known as the 'ironic process theory'.[4]

It's a simple concept: the harder you try *not* to think about something, the more you will think about it. I want you to try it right now. For the next ten seconds, do not, under any circumstances, think about a huge, pink elephant.

What are you thinking about? A huge, pink elephant, right?

The same thing happens with food. When you tell yourself, 'I am not allowed to eat chocolate,' your brain doesn't file this away as a helpful rule. Instead, it creates a mental obsession with chocolate. The restriction triggers your brain's rebellion mechanism – the more forbidden something becomes, the more irresistible it appears. The craving intensifies until it becomes an overwhelming compulsion that sweeps away your best intentions, often leading to consuming far more than you ever intended – sometimes to the point of physical discomfort.

This is the 'deprivation-binge' cycle, and it's a direct result of making certain foods forbidden.

A sustainable plan doesn't have a forbidden list, it has a strategy. By giving yourself permission to eat the foods you love, but within a smart, science-backed framework, you take away their power. The cake is no longer a forbidden, mystical object of desire. It's just cake. And you are an adult who can choose to enjoy it, or not, on your own terms.

## THE DEPRIVATION-BINGE CYCLE AND THE PSYCHOLOGY OF THE 'LAST MEAL'

The 'pink elephant' problem explains why you can't stop *thinking* about the forbidden food. But it doesn't quite explain the sheer ferocity of the urge that takes over when you finally give in: the feeling that you have to eat the *entire* packet, right now.

This isn't just a thought – it's a physiological takeover. To understand it fully, we need to look at what's really going on in your brain and your body.

When you live in a state of restriction, with a long list of 'bad' foods, you create a scarcity mindset. Any time you 'break a rule' and eat one of those forbidden foods, your primitive 'lizard brain' enters a state of panic. The 'lizard brain' – the amygdala and brain stem – is the oldest part of your brain, and it has been keeping humans alive for millions of years. It doesn't understand modern dieting; it only understands survival. When you restrict food, this ancient part of your brain interprets it as famine and goes into emergency mode.

Your 'CEO brain' – the prefrontal cortex – is the rational, logical part that can plan, make decisions, and think long-term. But when the lizard brain is in panic mode, it essentially hijacks your CEO brain's ability to make calm, sensible choices about food. It thinks, 'Oh my God, this is it! This is my only chance to eat this! I don't know when I'll be allowed it again, so I must eat all of it, as fast as I can, before the food police show up and take it away!'

This is the 'last meal' mentality. You're not eating for pleasure; you're eating out of fear. It's the same mindset that leads to the frantic, pre-diet binge on a Sunday night, where you try to eat every 'bad' thing in the house because you know that as of Monday it's off-limits. This scarcity mindset is a direct consequence of creating 'forbidden' foods, and it is the psychological driver of a binge.

## THE BIOLOGY OF THE REBOUND

Something is also happening on a hormonal level. Chronic restriction and dieting can lower the levels of leptin, your primary appetite and satiety hormone. Your body dials down this signal because it thinks a famine is underway and it wants you to stay hungry in order to seek out food. Then, if you eat the high-sugar, high-fat 'fun food', it lights up your brain's reward system like a Christmas tree, triggering a huge release of feel-good chemicals. But because your leptin signal is suppressed (through dieting), the 'stop' signal is weak, delayed or even non-existent.

Think about it: your brain is getting a massive, screaming 'GO!' signal from its reward pathways, but only a tiny, muffled 'stop' signal from its satiety hormones. It's like driving a car with the accelerator pushed to the floor and brakes made of sponge. You are biochemically programmed to keep going.

This is why you can eat an entire packet of biscuits and still not feel 'full', just sick. It is not a failure of your willpower. It is a predictable, logical, biological consequence of the restriction that came earlier. The four Ps method we have looked at already is the biological antidote to this destructive cycle. By giving yourself permission, you dismantle the 'last meal' panic, and by pairing your foods smartly, you support your satiety hormones, giving your body a functioning set of brakes.

## THE REMINDER: THE 4PS METHOD FOR FUN FOODS

Don't forget your simple, four-step checklist from chapter 4 for enjoying any tier 3 foods without the hormonal chaos or the emotional spiral.

### 1. PORTION: DECIDE YOUR DOSE

**The how:** Before you take the first bite, consciously decide on a sensible portion. This is the single most powerful act of control. You can have the cake, but you probably don't need the giant corner slice.

**The why:** By pre-committing to a portion size, you are using your wise, logical CEO brain to make a decision, before your impulsive lizard brain gets hijacked by the pleasure of the food itself.

### 2. PLANNING: TIMING IS EVERYTHING

**The how:** A planned dessert after a balanced dinner is a joyful, controlled experience. That same piece of cake eaten as a panicked, standalone snack at 4 p.m. when you're stressed and hungry is a recipe for disaster.

**The why:** Your hormonal state matters. When you are calm and already feeling satisfied from a good meal, you are making a choice from a place of pleasure. When you are stressed and your blood sugar is low, you are making a choice from a place of desperation.

## 3. PAIRING: NEVER EAT A FUN FOOD NAKED

**The how:** Never eat a sugary or starchy treat on an empty stomach. Always 'pair' it with a meal that is rich in protein and fibre.

**The why:** This is a direct application of the blood sugar science we learned in chapter 2. The protein and fibre from your main meal act as a buffer, slowing down the absorption of the sugar from your dessert. This dramatically reduces the glucose spike, preventing the subsequent crash and the hormonal hangover.

## 4. PACE: SAVOUR IT LIKE A PRO

**The how:** Eat it slowly. Put your fork down between bites. Pay attention to the texture, the flavour, the experience of eating it.

**The why:** When you eat mindfully, two things happen. First, you give your brain and stomach the 20 minutes they need for their fullness signals to kick in. Second, you will find you are satisfied with a much smaller amount. The pleasure is in the first few bites, not in mindless shovelling.

To understand how powerful this mindset shift is, let me tell you about my client, Sophia.

### SOPHIA'S STORY

The undisputed queen of the all-or-nothing cycle, Sophia's life was divided into two distinct, warring states: 'on the wagon' Sophia and 'off the wagon' Sophia.

'On the wagon' Sophia was a saint of deprivation. She would eat perfectly for weeks at a time, surviving on a joyless diet of steamed fish and plain vegetables. She would turn down every dinner invitation, avoid every social event and pack her own sad little Tupperware box for work lunches. She was getting results, but she was miserable, isolated and living in a fragile state of constant vigilance.

Then would come the inevitable 'off-the-wagon' moment. It was never a gentle step off: it was a cliff dive. A friend's wedding. A stressful week at work. One single, unplanned biscuit. That was all it took. The floodgates would open. 'Well, I've ruined it now,' her inner critic would scream, and she would proceed to eat her way through the weekend, in a haze of guilt due to all the sugary, carby food she was consuming.

Her rock bottom wasn't the food itself; it was the crushing weight of the shame she felt on Monday morning after an off-the-wagon weekend. It was the feeling of having to start the entire marathon all over again, from a starting line that seemed to recede each week.

Her turning point came before a planned holiday to Italy. She was filled with a sense of dread so profound it made her feel sick. 'I have two options,' she told me, her voice flat with resignation. 'I can either be the boring, difficult one who orders a plain salad in the land of pasta and doesn't drink the wine, and hate my entire holiday, or I can "let myself go", eat everything, and come back a stone heavier, hating myself. Which circle of hell should I choose?'

I told her there was a third option. An option where she could eat the pasta and drink the wine, and enjoy every single moment of

> her holiday without guilt or weight gain. And I introduced her to the four Ps method.
>
> I explained that her goal for the holiday was not to be 'good' or 'bad', but to practise being a discerning, mindful adult who was in control of her own pleasure.
>
> She was terrified. It went against every diet rule she had ever known. But she was desperate enough to try.
>
> She messaged me from a sun-drenched terrace in Tuscany a few days later. Sophia's words were so full of light it felt like a different person had written them. 'Last night,' she wrote, 'we went to this incredible little restaurant. I was so anxious. But I decided to try the four Ps. I ordered the grilled sea bass with roasted vegetables for my main [Pairing]. And then, I did something I haven't done in years: I looked at the dessert menu. I ordered the tiramisu [Planning]. When it arrived, I told myself I would have three perfect spoonfuls [Portion]. I ate them so slowly [Pace], savouring every single taste. It was the most delicious thing I have ever eaten. And then ... I put the spoon down. And I was done. I felt satisfied, not stuffed. I didn't spiral. I just had some of the dessert and moved on. This feels like witchcraft.'

Sophia's breakthrough wasn't just about the tiramisu. It was linked to the profound realisation that we don't have to live in the extremes of sainthood and sin. The four Ps method isn't a set of restrictions; it is our permission slip to live a normal, happy, delicious life without undoing all our progress.

## THE '100 PER CENT CONSISTENCY' MINDSET (AKA WHY THE 80/20 RULE IS A TRAP)

Sophia's story also dismantles one of the most persistent dieting myths: the 80/20 rule. You've probably heard it a million times:

'Just be "good" 80 per cent of the time, and you can be "bad" 20 per cent of the time.' It sounds balanced. It sounds reasonable. But it is a trap. The 80/20 rule keeps you locked in food jail. It perpetuates the language of 'good' and 'bad', of morality and sin. It frames your '20 per cent' – the slice of cake or the couple of biscuits – as a transgression, a cheat, a moment of weakness. It ensures that you will always feel a little bit guilty, even when you are following the 'rule'.

I want to propose a more powerful, more liberating idea. I don't want you to be 'good' 80 per cent of the time. Instead, I want you to be 100 per cent consistent.

Now, before you throw this book across the room, hear me out. I am not talking about being 100 per cent *perfect*. I am talking about being 100 per cent *consistent* with your new identity as someone who is a calm, conscious and empowered decision-maker around food.

Think about this in terms of your personal financial budget. A smart budget doesn't just have categories for rent, bills and groceries. It has a dedicated and guilt-free category for fun and entertainment – for the cinema, for meals out, for buying that new pair of shoes. When you spend money from your fun and entertainment category, are you 'cheating' on your budget? Are you being 'bad' with your money? Of course not. You are *following* your budget perfectly. The spending was planned, it was intentional, and it is a vital part of a sustainable, joyful financial life.

The four Ps method is how you create and manage the 'fun food' category in your life's budget. When you use the four Ps method to mindfully enjoy a slice of cake on your friend's birthday, you are not being part of a 20 per cent 'failure'; you are being 100 per cent consistent with your identity as a woman who enjoys life's pleasures strategically and without guilt. When you use the upcoming 'worth-it' filter (page 146) to politely decline a stale office biscuit, you are being 100 per cent consistent with your identity as a woman with high standards. When you have an off day and eat the whole tub of ice cream, and you practise self-compassion by getting right back on track with your next meal, you are being 100 per cent consistent with your identity as a resilient woman who learns from her experiences.

This is the ultimate mindset shift. There are no more 'good' days or 'bad' days. There are simply days where you are practising your new identity. Some days the practice will be messy. Some days it will be graceful. But you are always, 100 per cent of the time, the woman who is in charge.

## YOUR OUT-AND-ABOUT PLAYBOOK: A SOCIAL SURVIVAL GUIDE

The real test of the four Ps method often comes when you have to navigate the complex world of social eating. Here is your playbook for handling the most common scenarios with grace and confidence.

### 1. THE RESTAURANT DESSERT MENU

You've had a beautiful, balanced main course. The dessert menu arrives. Apply the four Ps. Suggest sharing one dessert between two (Portion) after eating your protein-rich meal (Pairing). Eat it slowly and savour it (Pace). It's a thought-through part of the meal (Planning).

### 2. THE CINEMA TRIP

The smell of popcorn is intoxicating. The old you would get the giant bucket. The new you eats a balanced dinner before you go (Pairing). You aim to buy the smallest size of popcorn (Planning and Portion) and eat it mindfully during the film (Pace).

## 3. THE OFFICE CAKE AMBUSH

It's 3 p.m. and someone brings in a cake to work. This is a danger zone as your blood sugar is likely at its lowest at this time. This is where you prepare your response (Planning). Make sure you finish your balanced lunch first (Pairing), and then make the decision to have just a small slice (Portion), whilst chatting with your colleagues (Pace).

> **CHOOSING YOUR INDULGENCE: THE WORTH-IT FILTER**
>
> 'How do I decide when to use the four Ps method and when to just say no?'
>
> This is a valid question. The goal is to elevate you from a passive, mindless consumer to a discerning connoisseur of your own pleasure. To do this, you will use a simple, powerful mental model called 'the worth-it filter'. Before you eat a tier 3 food, you will pause and ask two quick filter questions:
>
> **'Do I really, truly want this?'**
>
> This is the first gatekeeper. It helps you distinguish between a genuine desire and mindless eating. Are you craving this specific chocolate biscuit, or are you just eating it because it's on the plate in the middle of a boring meeting? Are you truly hungry, or are you just feeling stressed, bored or tired?
>
> **'Is this specific version of it worth it?'**
>
> This is the second, more sophisticated gatekeeper question. This is where you become a connoisseur. You might genuinely want a brownie. But is the dry, slightly stale,

mass-produced brownie from the office canteen worth it? Or, would you rather wait and have an incredible, warm, gooey, dark chocolate brownie from that amazing bakery you love, when you genuinely want it? Think about it: is *this* cheap, watery glass of house wine worth it? Or would you rather have one beautiful, expensive glass of your favourite red that you will truly savour?

The worth-it filter empowers you to say 'No, thank you,' to low-quality indulgences, not from a place of restriction, but from a place of high self-worth and impeccable standards. You're not dieting; you've just got better taste than to waste a pleasurable experience on something mediocre. It brings intention back to the forefront.

## 4. A GRACEFUL 'NO, THANK YOU'

This is the advanced level. What do you do when your friend, your colleague, or your lovely, well-meaning mother is actively trying to get you to eat more than you want? You need simple, polite, unbreakable scripts to counteract these situations.

**The scenario:** The 'Go on, just have one more!' friend.

**The script:** Smile warmly and say, 'Oh my God, it was absolutely amazing, but I am so perfectly, happily full right now. Honestly, another bite would spoil that! Please, you finish it.'

**Why it works:** It's overwhelmingly positive ('amazing', 'perfectly, happily full'). It's about *your* state, not their food. And it gives them permission to enjoy it.

**The scenario:** The person who shows love through food. They offer you a second giant slice of their famous lasagne.

**The script:** 'That was honestly the most delicious thing I've eaten all week. I'm so full right now, but could I possibly take a small piece home for my lunch tomorrow? I'd love to enjoy it again.'

**Why it works:** You are validating their effort and their love (the highest compliment). You are not rejecting their food; you are just deferring it. You are taking control of the Portion and Planning in a way that makes them feel appreciated, not refused.

## YOUR HORMONAL PLAYBOOK: HOW TO NAVIGATE YOUR LUTEAL PHASE CRAVINGS

For many women, the week before a period (the luteal phase) can feel like your body has been hijacked by the sugar gremlin. The cravings for carbs and chocolate can be overwhelming. This is not a failure of your willpower; it is a profound biological and hormonal event.

**The science:** As we've seen already, during your luteal phase, as progesterone rises, your insulin sensitivity can naturally decrease, making your blood sugar a little more volatile. At the same time, your levels of serotonin (the calming, feel-good neurotransmitter) can dip. Your body knows that eating carbohydrates is a very effective way to get more tryptophan (an amino acid) into the brain, which it then uses to make more serotonin. That intense craving for a chocolate bar is not just a craving for sugar; it's your brain's desperate, biological attempt to self-medicate and make itself feel better.

**The strategy:** Don't fight it; but feed it smarter. Instead of fighting this urge, we are going to honour it with better tools.

- **Upgrade your carb:** Your brain is asking for a tool. Instead of giving it a 'paper fire' carb like chocolate or biscuits (which will lead to a crash and make things worse), give it a 'slow log' carb. Strategically, increasing the size of your cupped-hand portion of smart carbs like sweet potato, quinoa or a baked potato with your evening meal can provide a gentler, more sustained serotonin boost but without the crash.
- **Make magnesium your best friend:** Magnesium is a powerful relaxation mineral that can be a game-changer for PMS symptoms. It's also found in one of the things you're probably craving: dark chocolate. A few squares of high-quality (70 per cent cocoa or higher) dark chocolate can be a brilliant tool here, as it provides magnesium and satisfies the chocolate craving. You can also try other magnesium-rich foods like almonds, pumpkin seeds and spinach.
- **Protein is non-negotiable:** Always apply the Pairing rule from the four Ps method. Ensure you have a solid palm of protein *before* you have your extra carbs. This is your ultimate insurance policy against a major blood sugar spike.

## LET'S TALK ABOUT ALCOHOL

Alcohol is the ultimate 'fun reward' for many of us. It's how we relax, socialise and treat ourselves. I am not going to tell you that you have to give up alcohol forever. But I must be honest with you about its impact.

As we learned in the sleep chapter, alcohol is a sedative that wrecks your sleep quality. It's also a source of empty calories, and it lowers your inhibitions, making you far more likely to make poor food choices ('drunk food' is a phenomenon for a reason).

Our goal is harm reduction. Here is the smart woman's guide to enjoying a drink.

- **Hydrate first:** Never drink on an empty stomach and a dehydrated system. Start with a large glass of mineralised water.
- **Choose your poison wisely:** Clear spirits like gin or vodka, accompanied by a sugar-free mixer (like soda water and fresh lime) are a much better choice from a blood sugar perspective than sugary cocktails, beer or sweet wines. (The tiny amount of natural sugar in the lime won't spike your blood sugar like cocktail mixers will.)
- **Apply the 90-minute rule:** As we've discussed, create a 90-minute buffer between your last sip of alcohol and your head hitting the pillow. This gives your liver a head start on metabolising it, lessening its impact on your deep sleep.

Here are some additional strategies for navigating social situations with alcohol while maintaining your health goals.

- **For parties and events:** Eat a protein-rich meal before drinking, alternate each alcoholic drink with water, and consider bringing your own mixer (sparkling water with fresh lime) so you're not limited to sugary options.
- **For holidays and celebrations:** Focus on the social connection rather than the drinks. You can still participate fully while being strategic about your choices – nurse one good-quality drink slowly rather than multiple lower-quality ones.
- **For weekends away:** Pack your own mixers and snacks so you're not dependent on whatever's available. Remember, you're in control of your choices, not restricted by them.

# YOUR SEVENTH ACTION PLAN: THE MINI 'FUN-FOOD' RITUAL

**The mindset shift:** A craving isn't a command – it's just information. You're the boss of your brain, not the other way around.

Here's the truth: there are no 'scary' foods, only foods you've been taught to fear through years of diet culture messaging. This week is about reclaiming your natural relationship with all types of food.

**The goal:** Normalise previously 'forbidden' foods by removing the moral weight you've attached to them.

**The task:** Choose one food that you've labelled as 'bad', 'unhealthy' or 'dangerous'. This might be chocolate, crisps, pastry or anything else you've put on the forbidden list.

## THIS WEEK'S PRACTICE

- **Planning:** Give yourself full permission to eat this food. Not as a 'treat' or 'cheat', but as a normal food choice that fits into your overall nourishment.
- **Pace:** When you choose to eat it, eat it mindfully. Sit down, pay attention to the taste, texture and how it makes you feel, both physically and emotionally.
- **Portion:** Serve yourself a reasonable amount on a proper plate or bowl. This isn't about restriction, it's about eating like a normal person rather than sneaking or bingeing.
- **Pairing:** Have it as part of a balanced-eating occasion. If it's chocolate, maybe after lunch. If it's crisps, perhaps with a sandwich. This supports stable blood sugar and satisfaction.

> What you might notice:
>
> - The food isn't as exciting when it's not forbidden.
> - You naturally want less when you know you can have it anytime.
> - The guilt and shame around the food starts to fade.
> - You can stop eating when satisfied rather than finishing everything.
>
> **Remember:** The goal isn't to eliminate these foods or prove you have willpower. It's to develop a calm, neutral relationship where all foods can fit into your life without drama.

You have the tools and the mindset to integrate pleasure into your life without the fear of the spiral. You have a plan for your nourishing meals and a strategy for your joyful extras.

Your food life is sorted. Now, it's time to build a body that is as strong and resilient as your new mindset. In the next chapter, we're going to talk about training – how to get incredible results and build a lean, toned physique without having to live at the gym.

# CHAPTER 8
# THE STRENGTH CODE

For years, you've maybe been the cardio queen. The woman who's 'just been for a run'. The one sweating through spin classes, grinding through high-intensity interval training (HIIT) sessions, treating the treadmill like it owes you money. You've done everything the fitness industry told you to do: burned thousands of calories, sweated buckets. And yet, here you are, exhausted, hungry all the time, and looking pretty much the same as you did three years ago.

Frustrating, isn't it?

Here's what nobody tells you: all that cardio might be making you fatter. Not directly, but hear me out. Every hour you spend on a treadmill is like working an hourly job – you clock in, burn some calories, clock out, and then need do it all over again tomorrow. The moment you stop, so do the benefits.

Strength training, on the other hand? That's like building an investment portfolio. Every bit of muscle you build works for you 24/7, burning calories while you sleep, while you work, while you're sitting on the sofa watching Netflix. It's the difference between renting and owning: one requires constant payment; the other builds equity alongside paying the mortgage.

## THE UNEXPLAINED SCIENCE: TRAINING FOR THE FEMALE BODY

Let's break down what's happening in your body when you do all that cardio. Every time you go for an hour-long run, your body floods with cortisol – the stress hormone that makes you hold on to belly fat like it's a prized possession. Your body thinks you're running from danger. Every single day.

So, what does it do in response? It slows down your metabolism to conserve energy (clearly there's an emergency somewhere if you're running this much), holds on to fat (especially around your middle), and breaks down muscle tissue for fuel. You're literally eating your own muscles.

Meanwhile, your friend who lifts weights three times a week but couldn't run for a bus? She's got a metabolism that's absolutely flying because she's built muscle tissue, which burns calories around the clock.

Think about it another way: imagine your metabolism is a fire. Cardio is like throwing paper on the fire – quick burst of flames, then nothing. Strength training is like adding proper logs – they burn slower but for much longer, keeping the fire going all day and night.

## WHY YOUR HORMONES MATTER MORE THAN YOUR WORKOUT

If you're a woman, especially if you're between 30 and 50 years old, we need to have a serious chat about why generic fitness advice is failing you.

We start with a stark fact: most commonly held 'rules' for exercise were designed for men's bodies.

But women's bodies don't operate on a 24-hour cycle like a man's; they operate on an approximate 28-day cycle, and this changes everything about how you should train.

During the first half of your cycle (power phase: from your period to ovulation), your oestrogen rises. An anabolic hormone, it helps you build muscle and recover faster. Your body is primed for strength gains during this phase. You're basically on natural steroids (legal ones, don't worry).

But, during the second half of your cycle (luteal phase: from ovulation to your period), progesterone takes over. It is a catabolic hormone, meaning it can break down muscle tissue. Your core body temperature is also higher, making everything feel harder, and you're more insulin resistant, too, which is why you crave carbs like mad during this time.

So, when some unknowing personal trainer tells you to 'push through' when you're in week four of your cycle and feeling like death, you now know to ignore them.

### THE SMART APPROACH TO FITNESS

Remember, work with your biology, not against it.

In your power phase (weeks 1 and 2 of your cycle), push for new personal bests. Go for heavier weights. Add that extra rep. This is when you should focus on applying progressive overload (gradually challenging your muscles more each session to force adaptation and growth).

In your luteal phase (weeks 3 and 4 of your cycle), be smart and listen to your body. Focus on excellent form, maybe lower the weight slightly and increase the reps, but really tune into the mind-muscle connection. Also try more restorative activities like yoga and walking. Add to this the concept of the 'deload week'.

> The deload week is the week of your period (or the week just before, if that's when you feel your worst). Still work out, but intentionally reduce the intensity. Cut the weight you're lifting by about 30 to 40 per cent and stop each set well short of failure. The goal is movement and recovery, not intensity. This strategic rest is not a weakness; it's an intelligent decision that will allow you to hit your next 'power phase' feeling strong and refreshed, instead of burned out.

## THE HORMONAL GAME-CHANGER

For women dealing with hormone challenges – whether that's PCOS, perimenopause, thyroid issues or just the monthly rollercoaster of your cycle – strength training isn't just helpful, it's transformative. Here's the science.

- **Insulin sensitivity magic:** Every time you lift weights, your muscles become glucose vacuum cleaners. They can pull sugar from your bloodstream more efficiently, which means your body needs less insulin to manage blood sugar. Lower insulin levels mean less hormone chaos across the board.
- **Stress hormone regulation:** Strength training helps regulate cortisol – your stress hormone that loves to store fat around your middle and mess with your sleep. Unlike endless cardio (which can actually increase cortisol), progressive weight training gives you the stress-busting benefits without the hormone disruption.
- **Metabolic hormone boost:** Building muscle tissue increases your metabolic rate and improves how your body processes nutrients. More muscle means better thyroid function, more

stable energy, and improved regulation of hunger hormones like leptin and ghrelin.
- **Real-world results:** I spent years doing cardio and feeling exhausted. Three months of proper strength training? My energy stabilised, my mood improved, and my body finally started responding to good nutrition. My doctor was impressed. I wasn't surprised.

This isn't wellness influencer nonsense. This is biochemistry. For women's complex hormone systems, building muscle creates a foundation that supports everything else – from cycle regulation to stress management to sustainable fat loss.

### CLAIRE'S STORY

Claire, a 45-year-old marketing manager was, in her own words, 'addicted to cardio'. She ran five days a week, clocking up over 20 miles, and religiously attended two spin classes on the weekend. She was working incredibly hard. She was also exhausted, constantly hungry and deeply frustrated.

'I'm running all the time,' she told me. 'I'm burning thousands of calories. So why am I not losing weight? If anything, I feel ... softer.'

Claire was trapped in the 'hourly job' mindset. Her endless cardio was keeping her cortisol levels high, which was encouraging her body to store fat and making her feel ravenous. She was running on empty. The advice I gave her was to stop running for four weeks and trade her seven weekly cardio sessions for just three 45-minute, full-body strength workouts.

She was terrified. 'But I'll get fat!' she said. 'I won't be burning any calories!'

I asked her to trust the process. The first two weeks were a mental battle. She felt lazy. But then, things started to change. She

> wasn't as hungry. Her sleep improved. At the end of the four weeks, her weight had barely changed, but her photos told a different story. Her waist was smaller. Her arms had shape. Her posture was better.
>
> 'I'm working out less than half of what I was before,' she told me, 'and my body has changed more than it has in years. It feels like I've found a cheat code.'
>
> Claire hadn't found a shortcut. She had just switched from being an hourly worker to a smart investor.

## THE ONLY EXERCISES YOU'LL EVER NEED

The world of strength training can feel overwhelming, but it all boils down to just five fundamental human movements. Master these patterns, and you'll have the keys to the kingdom. Here's your practical template to build confidence and results.

For anyone unsure as to the exercises – how they look, how they're done – you can scan the QR code and it'll take you to some reels where I show you how to do them correctly and efficiently.

**EXERCISE ABBREVIATIONS:**

- DL = Deadlift (hip hinge movement)
- BW = Bodyweight (no added weight)
- DB = Dumbbell
- BB = Barbell

## YOUR COMPLETE WORKOUT TEMPLATE

**Frequency:** 2–3 times per week
**Duration:** 20–30 minutes
**Rest:** 48 hours between sessions

## THE FIVE ESSENTIAL MOVEMENT PATTERNS

### 1. Squat pattern (sit and stand)
**What it does:** Builds legs, glutes and core. Essential for daily life.
**BEGINNER:** Bodyweight chair squats
**INTERMEDIATE:** Goblet squats (hold dumbbell to chest)
**ADVANCED:** Barbell back squats
**Sets and reps:** 2–3 sets of 8–12 reps

### 2. Hinge pattern (picking things up)
**What it does:** Strengthens your entire back side – glutes, hamstrings, lower back.
**BEGINNER:** Glute bridges
**INTERMEDIATE:** Dumbbell deadlifts
**ADVANCED:** Barbell deadlifts
**Sets and reps:** 2–3 sets of 6–10 reps

### 3. Push pattern (upper body strength)
**What it does:** Builds chest, shoulders, triceps and core stability.
**BEGINNER:** Wall push-ups or knee push-ups
**INTERMEDIATE:** Full push-ups
**ADVANCED:** Weighted push-ups or overhead press
**Sets and reps:** 2–3 sets of 5–15 reps (adjust to your level)

### 4. Pull pattern (posture power)

**What it does:** Fixes desk posture, builds a strong back, creates waist definition.

**BEGINNER:** Resistance band rows
**INTERMEDIATE:** Dumbbell bent-over rows
**ADVANCED:** Pull-ups or barbell rows
**Sets and reps:** 2–3 sets of 8–12 reps

### 5. Core pattern (stability and protection)

**What it does:** Protects your spine, improves posture, builds deep core strength.

**BEGINNER:** Wall plank or knee plank
**INTERMEDIATE:** Full plank
**ADVANCED:** Plank variations (side plank, plank up-downs)
**Sets and reps:** 2–3 sets of 15–60 seconds

## YOUR WEEKLY WORKOUT TEMPLATE

### WORKOUT A: Full body foundation

Squat pattern – 3 sets
Push pattern – 2 sets
Pull pattern – 3 sets
Core pattern – 2 sets

### WORKOUT B: Power and stability

Hinge pattern – 3 sets
Pull pattern – 2 sets
Squat pattern – 2 sets
Core pattern – 3 sets

***Schedule options (following days of the week):***
Beginner: (Workout) A, Rest, B, Rest, Rest, A, Rest
Intermediate: (Workout) A, Rest, B, Rest, A, Rest, B

## THE SYSTEM: YOUR THREE-PHASE WORKOUT PLAN

What follows is a flexible workout blueprint for the real world. The three stages of this system offer ideas of how to train to build up both your confidence and your strength. This is all about building a workout routine that works for you in the real world, with the natural cycle of your body.

The most common thing to happen is to take on an all-or-nothing mentality with training. If you've not lifted a weight in years, you need to build up the habit slowly. So, this is your gameplan.

### PHASE 1: WEEKS 1–2

***Building the habit***
**Goal**: Establishing consistency.

Over these two weeks you're going to show up three times a week. That's it. You're going to complete three workouts, and they can be the same exact ones each time if that's what you're comfortable with. We're just focusing on building the habit here, not variety. Don't worry about hitting certain muscle groups just yet, we're just turning up and doing the movements.

Always, but particularly over these two weeks, ensure to properly warm up for five minutes before getting started. This can be any sort of light movement until you feel nice and warm – it can be a jog on the spot or star jumps.

Look at your workout template above to get ideas on what you can do. Make a note of what you're planning on doing each time so you can stick to it without having to think about it on the spot. Pick five exercises and do three sets of 8–12 repetitions (reps). If using them, go for lighter weights.

We're not looking at perfect form or heavy weights in this stage, nor do we want to log our progress or investigate it too closely. We just want to get into the habit of turning up and moving.

## PHASE 2: WEEKS 3–7

### *Baseline and Progression*

**Goal:** Track progress and understand your body's patterns.

You've done two weeks of sticking to your schedule and getting yourself into the habit of turning up. You're slowly gaining confidence in your space – whether that's a gym mat in your living room or the gym floor – so we need to start looking at how to build on it in a way that lets you keep it up, realistically.

You're going to do the same thing as you did in weeks 1 and 2 – turn up three times a week, pick five exercises and do three sets of 8–12 reps each. But you're now going to make a note of what you're doing, too. Using a notepad or your notes app on your phone, take note of the weights you used in each exercise and how many repetitions you managed. If you felt anything whilst completing the exercises, make note of that, too – did you feel a twinge? Did you feel that your form needs improving? Did you feel more tired this time around completing a particular exercise?

Making note of it all allows you to look into it next time and allows you to start noticing patterns in the long term. You'll start to recognise that being in a different part of your cycle affects your strength and energy, or that when your schedule is a bit busier at work, you're more tired than on the weekend, when you usually get the chance for more rest in the morning.

## A SUGGESTED WORKOUT LOG

Date: _____ Workout Type: _____

| Exercise | Weight | Set 1 Reps | Set 2 Reps | Set 3 Reps | RPE* Score |
|---|---|---|---|---|---|
| _____ | ____kg | ____ | ____ | ____ | ___/10 |
| _____ | ____kg | ____ | ____ | ____ | ___/10 |
| _____ | ____kg | ____ | ____ | ____ | ___/10 |
| _____ | ____kg | ____ | ____ | ____ | ___/10 |
| _____ | ____kg | ____ | ____ | ____ | ___/10 |

Notes: _____

\* Rate of perceived exertion – see Rate of perceived exertion box on page 168.

All this data becomes your baseline for improvement and allows you to progress your workouts, adding variety and new challenges to keep you interested.

- **Weeks 3 – 4:** Learn the movements, focus on form.
- **Weeks 5 – 6:** Add weight, or increase repetitions.
- **Week 7:** Move to the next difficulty level on your exercises. For example, if you've been doing planks on your knees, have a go at a full plank and see how it feels.

Exercise is something that you should keep building slowly over time. Over these seven weeks, we want to get into the routine of doing this, but long term, you can take your time moving through phases depending on how you're feeling month to month. It's not about rushing through the process but about setting a habit in place and making it work for your own life and routines.

## HOW TO WIN EVERY WEEK

Aim to gradually improve over time – this might mean one extra rep this week, a small weight increase next week, or simply maintaining good form for all your sets. Progress isn't always linear, and that's perfectly normal. Some weeks you'll improve, others you'll maintain, and occasionally you might even need to scale back if you're tired or stressed. This is called progressive overload, and consistency over time is what guarantees long-term progress.

Your log book turns your fitness into a game you can't lose. Your only opponent each week is you from last week. Let's say you do the same workout. You open your logbook and see your numbers from last week. Your goal is simply to beat them, even by a tiny margin.

For example, last Monday, for the goblet squat, you did 10kg for 12, 10, 8 reps. This week, maybe you manage 10kg for 12, 11, 8 reps. That is a win. You did one more rep. You are officially stronger.

For the dumbbell deadlift, you hit 12 reps on your first two sets with 12kg. This is a sign! It's time to go up in weight. The next week, maybe you try the 14kg dumbbells and you get 14kg for 9, 8, 8 reps. The number of reps is lower, but you lifted a heavier weight. That is a massive win.

Seeing your progress written down is such a powerful source of motivation. It is undeniable proof that the work you are doing is making a difference. It shows you are getting stronger.

The secret to making progress is simply doing very slightly more than last time. That's it. That's the whole secret.

It's called progressive overload, and it's the only way to guarantee progress.

## PHASE 3: WEEKS 7–12

### *Intelligent progression*
**Goal:** Apply progressive overload strategically, based on your cycle.

Sometimes it can feel like your cycle is working against you when you're doing exercise. Your hormonal fluctuations over your cycle can have a deep effect on your energy and strength levels. You'll feel stronger when your oestrogen and testosterone levels are high in the first half of your cycle (follicular and ovulatory phases), and often weaker and more tired when your progesterone and oestrogen levels start to drop in the second half (luteal and menstrual phases). Rather than pushing through these as if nothing has changed and demotivating yourself, we need to start working with our bodies.

You've been tracking your progress in phase 2 – you've made a note of how workouts felt week to week and what was going on at the time, both in terms of your work and social life, and your cycle. You'll now know on which weeks you felt great and energetic, and when you've felt like your usual workout was like pulling teeth.

You're now going to start working with your body so you can leave the gym feeling good and motivated each time. By doing so, you're more likely to stick to your habit, rather than taking two weeks off when your hormones are just doing what they need to be doing.

## POWER WEEKS (DAYS 1–14 OF YOUR CYCLE / FOLLICULAR AND OVULATORY PHASES)

These are the weeks you're going to challenge yourself – you've got some extra strength and energy from your body's natural cycle, so we're going to use it. You're going to push for some new personal records – go up an extra weight for your exercises or do some additional repetitions. If you're feeling a proper boost, you can add an extra set of a completely new exercise to add variety. Use the extra motivation to explore.

## MAINTENANCE WEEK (DAYS 15–22 OF YOUR CYCLE / LUTEAL PHASE)

We're not looking for a challenge here. The plan this week is to maintain the current weights you played around with in your power weeks. You're going to focus your energy on perfecting your form rather than trying new things or adding to your workout routine. Listen to your body – if you feel yourself getting exhausted quickly, take it slow or reduce your weights. It's more important to complete a workout safely and maintain energy to still turn up to your next session, rather than work your way to complete exhaustion.

## DELOAD WEEK (DAYS 19–28 OF YOUR CYCLE / MENSTRUAL PHASE)

Your main focus this week is to show up and move gently. We're not looking at trying to beat any personal records. It's also going to realistically not be a week where you'll be able to maintain the same weights or repetitions you used in your luteal phase, and that's to be expected. Rather than trying to push through a workout you can't complete, or risk injuring yourself, make slight adjustments. Reduce any weights you're using by 20 to 30 per cent or ditch them altogether for light bodyweight exercises, if that feels better.

Focus on the quality of your movement here over anything else. Do some gentle yoga instead or go for a walk. Honour your body's need for rest and view it as a necessary part of your month. Rest is productive, not lazy.

Remember, for every part of the process, this isn't about obliteration and completely exhausting yourself. It's about movement. It's about keeping the promise to yourself and casting a vote for your new identity. It's about keeping it consistent in a way that fits in with a real life.

> **TAKING YOUR WORKOUTS TO THE NEXT LEVEL**
>
> Within these 12 weeks you've established a strong habit and should start feeling stronger and more confident in your exercising. You know your way around a gym mat and how you feel exercising different parts of your body, so start looking at different elements and parts of your body to start structuring your workout. If you feel up for it, some weeks you can add in an extra session or two. We're taking note of what works and feels good to you over these 12 weeks, so play around with your schedule and see what sticks.
>
> - **Upper body workouts:** Focus on chest, back, shoulders, arms (e.g. push-ups, rows, overhead press)
> - **Lower body workouts:** Focus on legs and glutes (e.g. squats, deadlifts, lunges)
> - **Full body workouts:** Include movements for both upper and lower body in one session.
>
> Weekly structure options:
>
> - **3 days/week:** 1 upper + 1 lower + 1 full body
> - **4 days/week:** 2 upper + 2 lower
> - **5 days/week:** 3 lower + 2 upper

## REDEFINING A 'SUCCESSFUL' WORKOUT

A word of warning: while your logbook is a powerful tool, it can also become a trap. You might look at your numbers from last week and feel pressure to beat them, every single time.

So what happens on the days you can't? What about when you've had a terrible night's sleep, or you're pre-menstrual, or you've had a draining day at work and you get to the gym and the weights just feel too heavy? What happens when you can't lift more or do that extra rep?

For the perfectionist in you, this can feel like failure. It can feel like you're going backwards. It's the kind of experience that can make you want to stop tracking, or even quit working out.

But progress isn't always linear. Sometimes, especially in weeks three and four of your cycle, the same weight can feel impossibly heavy. That's not failure – that's biology. Be aware of where you are in your menstrual cycle, and track your effort level as well as your weights.

To measure this, we can use a simple mental tool called the rate of perceived exertion (RPE). It's a scale of 1 to 10 that measures how hard a set felt to you, personally, on that specific day. Simply rate your workout using the scale below:

### RATE OF PERCEIVED EXERTION

- **RPE 1:** Sitting on the sofa

to

- **RPE 7:** The weight is challenging, you're working, but you're confident you have a few more good reps in the tank.

> - **RPE 9:** That was seriously hard. The last rep was a real grind, and you might have had one more perfect rep left in you, but that's it.
> - **RPE 10:** Absolute failure. You couldn't have done another rep even if you'd been offered a million pounds.
>
> For most of our workouts, the goal is to be working in that RPE 7 to 9 sweet spot.

Now, here is my final secret. Progress is not about the number on the dumbbell; it's about your RPE score. On a great day, when you're well rested and full of energy, lifting a 12kg dumbbell for your goblet squat might feel like an RPE 8. On a bad day, when you're tired, stressed and in your luteal phase, lifting that same 12kg dumbbell might feel like an RPE 10.

Did you fail on that second day because you didn't lift more weight? Absolutely not. In fact, you could argue you worked even harder. You still achieved the right stimulus for your muscles because the RPE was high. You still sent the signal to your body to adapt and get stronger. That is a successful workout.

This is how we untangle our self-worth from our performance. This new definition of a win is not just about beating the numbers. Instead, a successful workout is about showing up and giving the best effort you have available on that specific day. Sometimes, the biggest win is just getting through the door, moving your body with good form and hitting an RPE 8 when you felt like a 2.

> **MAKE IT STICK: BUILDING THE HABIT OF STRENGTH**
>
> - **The tiny habit:** Your only goal for each week is to complete one of your planned workouts. Just one. That's it. This builds a feeling of success and momentum.
> - **The environment tweak:** The night before a planned workout, lay out your gym kit, fill your water bottle, and put your gym bag by the door. This visual cue makes the decision to go almost automatic.
> - **The if–then plan:** '*If* I feel unmotivated before a workout, *then* I will just put my kit on and do the 3-minute warm-up.' (Spoiler: you'll almost never stop after that. Starting is the hardest part.)

## OVERCOMING GYMTIMIDATION

Knowing the plan is one thing. Walking into a busy gym and doing it is another. Here are some suggestions to make it feel less terrifying.

- **Go on a reccy:** Your first trip to a new gym is not a workout. Go at a quiet time. Your only job is to walk around, find the dumbbells, understand the gym equipment.
- **Create a safe zone:** For your first few workouts, it's okay to stick to your 'safe zone'. Pick a spot in the corner of the dumbbell area. You can get a phenomenal workout with just dumbbells.
- **The 'what to wear' question:** Wear something that makes you feel comfortable and confident, not something you think you *should* wear. No one cares if you have the latest matching gym set. They care even less if you don't. Comfort is king.

- **Headphones are your superpower:** They create an invisible shield that says, 'I'm in my world.' Put on a playlist that makes you feel like a badass.
- **Remember the truth:** Nobody is watching you. I promise. They are all too busy worrying about themselves.

## COMMON MISTAKES THAT KEEP YOU STUCK (AND HOW TO FIX THEM)

**Mistake:** 'Chasing soreness.' Thinking that if you're not cripplingly sore the next day, the workout wasn't effective.

**The fix:** Delayed onset muscle soreness (DOMS) is just a sign of a new stimulus. As you get fitter, you will become less sore. A little stiffness is the goal. Crippling soreness is a sign you overdid it and will compromise your next workout. (See more about DOMS on the next page.)

**Mistake:** 'Programme hopping.' Doing a different random workout every time you go to the gym.

**The fix:** You can't apply progressive overload if you're always doing something new. Stick to the same core exercises for at least 4 to 6 weeks to see real, measurable progress.

**Mistake:** 'Fearing the space.' Feeling like you don't 'belong' in the weights area.

**The fix:** You pay the same membership fee as the massive guy grunting in the corner. You have just as much right to be there as he does. Walk in with your plan, put your headphones on and own your space.

# SORENESS VS PAIN: A CRUCIAL DISTINCTION

As you start strength training, you will experience new sensations in your body. Some are good, productive and a sign of progress. Others might be warning signals. Learning to tell the difference is a vital skill.

## 1. DOMS (DELAYED ONSET MUSCLE SORENESS)

**What it is:** That achy, stiff feeling you get 1 to 2 days after a workout – you know, when you're moving like you're about 90 years old after leg day …

**What it means:** Your muscles are doing exactly what they're supposed to do. You've created tiny tears that your body will repair, making your muscles stronger. It's not damage – it's progress.

**What to do about it:** Don't just lie on the sofa feeling sorry for yourself. Move gently: a walk or some stretching. Or use a foam roller (using a long cylindrical roller to apply pressure to muscles – most gyms have them). This gets the blood flowing and speeds up recovery and it may help reduce muscle tension and improve flexibility, though the research on its recovery benefits is still developing. The pressure helps increase blood flow to the area, which can feel good and may aid recovery.

**The mindset:** As you get fitter, you'll get less DOMS from the same workout. That's good – it means you're adapting. To feel a bit stiff is the goal; feeling like you've been hit by a truck means you overdid it.

## 2. PAIN: 'SOMETHING FEELS WRONG'

**What it is:** Pain is completely different from muscle soreness. We're talking sharp, shooting, stabbing sensations that make you go 'Ow!' Usually in a joint like your knee, shoulder or lower back rather than the muscle itself, if it gets worse when you move or you feel it during an exercise, that's your body screaming at you to stop.

**What it means:** This is your body's alarm system sounding. It's not the good ache of muscles working, it's a warning that something's wrong. Could be you let your form slip, the weight's too heavy or you're about to injure yourself more seriously.

**What to do about it:** Stop. Right now. Don't be that person who thinks they can push through sharp pain because their ego's writing cheques their body can't cash. Drop the weight, check your form or pick a different exercise. Pushing through pain is the fastest way to end up on the sidelines for weeks or months.

**The mindset:** Learning the difference between good muscle ache and a warning pain is one of the most important skills you can develop. In the first case your muscles are having a chat with you, in the second they are screaming at you. Listen to both.

## YOUR EIGHTH ACTION PLAN: START BUILDING YOUR STRENGTH BANK

**The mindset shift:** Complete this sentence out loud: 'I am the type of person who ...' and fill in the blank with one healthy behaviour you've been practising. Say it like you mean it. You're not aspirational anymore – you're actual.

**The task:** Grab any notebook. Write 'My Strength Sessions' on the first page. This is now your workout log – track what you lift, how it felt and what you want to improve next time.

Now open your calendar. Block out three 45-minute slots this week.

**The action:** Label them 'Strength Training' and treat them like non-negotiable appointments. You wouldn't skip a meeting with your boss, don't skip meetings with your future self. Log these session – and off you go!

You now have the why, the what and the how of building a strong, metabolically active body. You have a flexible plan that can weather any storm. But how do we make these powerful workouts even *more* efficient? Time to learn how to get maximum results from every minute you spend exercising.

# CHAPTER 9
# THE TRAINING MINDSET SHIFT

Let's play 'Spot the Difference'. Here are two scenarios.

## *Scenario A*

It's Tuesday evening. You leave work late, sit in traffic for 25 minutes, then finally get to the gym. You spend 10 minutes changing into your kit. Hit the gym, do a set, then during your 'rest' time you check work emails. Read a passive-aggressive message from your boss. Heart rate spikes. Spend three minutes crafting a polite-but-firm response. Another set. More resting, but this time you get sucked into Instagram for five minutes, leaving you feeling inadequate. An hour and a half later, you've done about 30 minutes of actual training. Rush home knackered to sort out dinner and life.

## *Scenario B*

It's Tuesday evening. You leave work, and go straight home. Change into your gym kit, go to the living room, activate playlist, and put your phone on airplane mode. For 40 minutes, you're a focused machine, moving with purpose from exercise to exercise. You're sweaty, breathless and done. The same amount of training has been achieved as Scenario A but in less than half the time, plus you are already at home, feeling powerful and accomplished.

How did you get on? Did you spot the difference?

For years, you've been living in the exhausting world of Scenario A. You've been told a 'proper' workout must be long. More time equals better results, right?

This (incorrect) belief is the single biggest barrier standing between busy, high-achieving people and the bodies they want. It creates a false choice: either you sacrifice a 90-minute chunk of your evening to exercise, or you do nothing at all. And on most days, 'nothing at all' is the only realistic option.

This chapter introduces you to the liberating world of Scenario B. This is what I call the 40-minute metabolism multiplier – a strategic approach that maximizes workout density to create maximum metabolic stress in minimum time. Instead of spending 90 minutes in the gym, you get superior results in 40 focused minutes.

We're going to dismantle the myth that duration equals results. I'm going to show you how to productively increase your workout density (how much work you do in any given period) and intensity, but with no increase to the time taken to achieve this.

Intensity simply means how challenging the exercise feels to you personally – it's your subjective experience of effort during movement. Think of it as your internal effort meter: a gentle walk might feel like 3 out of 10 on your intensity scale, while sprinting upstairs might hit 9 out of 10. The beauty of intensity is that it's completely personal – what feels intense for you today might feel easier next month as you get stronger.

Welcome to efficient training: a practical approach that fits into busy schedules while still delivering meaningful results.

## THE SCIENCE: THE POWER OF WORKOUT DENSITY

Walk into any commercial gym and you'll see the enemy of progress: wasted time. Someone does a set, then sits on the bench for five minutes, scrolling through their phone. They are spending significantly more time resting than they are working. Their workout 'density' is incredibly low. Workout density is simply how much work you do in any given period. By strategically reducing our rest time, we can dramatically increase our density. This does more than just save time; it creates a powerful biological response called metabolic stress.

The metabolic stress response is one of the key drivers of muscle growth and fat loss. When you create this intense metabolic environment in your muscles, you're essentially forcing your body to adapt by building lean muscle tissue and ramping up your metabolism for hours after your workout ends.

Muscle growth is triggered by three main factors:

- **Mechanical tension:** Lifting heavy weights.
- **Muscle damage:** The tiny micro-tears we've talked about.
- **Metabolic stress:** This is the burning, fatigued sensation you feel in your muscles when they're working hard – such as when your legs feel wobbly during the last few squats, or your arms start shaking during push-ups. This muscle fatigue signals to your body to adapt and grow stronger.

The 'pump' isn't just muscles looking good, it's the feeling of them releasing these 'exercise molecules'. A 40-minute, high-density training session isn't just better for fat loss – it's a therapeutic treatment for your entire body and brain.

> **THE HORMONAL POWER OF THE 'PUMP'**
>
> The satisfying, swollen feeling (the 'pump') created in your muscles after a great workout is not just cosmetic. When muscles contract under intense stress, they release powerful proteins called myokines into your bloodstream.
>
> No gentle cardio session could ever replicate the three key effects caused by these 'exercise molecules'.
>
> - Powerful anti-inflammatory response.
> - Improved insulin sensitivity.
> - Mood-boosting, stress-reducing effects on your brain.

## TRAINING VS EXERCISING

Before we learn the techniques for the 40-minute metabolism multiplier, we need to make a crucial mental shift. For years, you've been 'exercising'. Often driven not by a feeling of pleasure but of obligation, exercising is showing up, going through the motions, watching the clock, keeping one eye on how others see you and the other on the calorie counter on the equipment screen.

Today, we are going to start 'training' instead.

Training means showing up with a clear plan. Every minute has purpose. You're focused, intentional and there for specific results. We're not there to 'burn calories' but to send powerful signals to our body to build muscle and to get stronger.

The key difference isn't how much you sweat, it's the quality of your attention during the session. Working out with intensity doesn't mean screaming and throwing weights around. It's acting with a quiet, focused energy. The concentration you put into that final grinding rep. How deliberately you control the weight. Most importantly, what you do during rest periods in between reps. The person who scrolls Instagram during her rest – she's just exercising. The person who is *training* uses that time strategically instead – focusing on breathing, sipping water, mentally rehearsing the next set or visualising the perfect form.

To help you step into the new identity of someone who trains, we are going to use a simple but powerful tool called 'bookending' – a 60-second ritual to start your workout, and a 60-second ritual to end it. These are your non-negotiable mental boundaries.

## THE 'CLOCKING IN' BOOKEND

Before you do anything, stand still for 60 seconds. Phone away. Eyes closed. Three deep breaths. Set one intention: for example, 'Focus on form,' or 'Push myself on final reps' – whatever feels right. This draws a line under your day's chaos and signals a focused state.

## THE 'CLOCKING OUT' BOOKEND

After your final set, stand still again. Eyes closed. Take three grateful breaths. Acknowledge one thing you did well: 'Went up in weight,' or 'Showed up when I didn't feel like it,' perhaps. This builds self-trust and reinforces the identity of someone who keeps promises to themselves.

This is how you transform your workout from a mindless chore into a mindful, empowering practice.

## MAKING YOUR WORKOUTS MORE EFFECTIVE

### WEAPON 1: THE SUPERSET

Our first and most powerful tool for increasing intensity is the superset. It's simple: you perform two different exercises back-to-back with minimal to no rest in between. The secret is to pair exercises that work opposing muscle groups.

This is more than just a time-saver; it's a performance enhancer. While one muscle group is working, the opposite muscle group is being actively stretched and relaxed. This can encourage you to perform more reps or lift slightly heavier weights on the next set. You're not just saving time; you're getting stronger, faster.

Plus, by eliminating most of the rest time, you keep your heart rate elevated for the entire workout. This dramatically increases the 'afterburn effect', meaning your metabolism stays up for hours after you've left the gym. You can turn a 40-minute workout into a metabolic advantage.

Superset example:

**Goblet squats (legs) paired with push-ups (upper body)**
- 12 squats then straight into 10 push-ups, then rest 90 seconds.
- Repeat for 3 rounds.

You've done the same work as separate exercises but in two-thirds of the time, with better metabolic benefits.

### WEAPON 2: THE FINISHER

A short, intense 3- to 5-minute burst at the end of your strength session. The aim is to completely empty the tank and spike your metabolism, forcing your body into working overtime for hours afterwards.

## THE TRAINING MINDSET SHIFT

*Your finisher protocol menu (choose one)*

- **The dumbbell thruster challenge:** Holding two light dumbbells at your shoulders, do a squat. As you stand up, press the dumbbells overhead. Do as many as you can in 3 minutes.
- **The dumbbell thruster intervals:** Hold two dumbbells at shoulder height. Set a timer for 5 minutes. Do 8 thrusters (squat down, stand up and press dumbbells overhead) at the top of every minute. The rest of the minute is your recovery.
- **The bodyweight burnout (aka Tabata):** Set a timer for 4 minutes. Do 20 seconds of burpees, followed by 10 seconds of rest. Repeat 8 times.

> **WHAT IS TABATA?**
>
> Tabata is a form of high-intensity interval training that alternates between 20 seconds of maximum effort and 10 seconds of rest for 4 minutes total. It's named after Dr Izumi Tabata, who proved this specific timing creates massive metabolic benefits in minimal time.

Long-rest workouts are great for mechanical tension. But shorter-rest, high-density workouts are brilliant for creating metabolic stress. Think of it like this: a long workout is like slow-cooking a stew. It works, but it takes hours. A high-density, 40-minute workout is like using a pressure cooker. You dramatically speed up the 'cooking' time by increasing the intensity and pressure inside the pot.

This is exactly what the 40-minute metabolism multiplier does. It's a strategic approach that maximises workout density to create maximum metabolic stress in minimum time. Instead of spending 90 minutes in the gym with long rest periods, you compress the same muscle-building and fat-burning stimulus into 40 focused minutes.

## BUILD YOUR FIRST 40-MINUTE METABOLISM MULTIPLIER

This takes your existing weekly workout template and transforms it using the superset and density principles we've just learned about.

**Warm-up** (5 minutes)

**Superset A** (3 rounds, 90-second rest between rounds)
- A1: Goblet squat (10–12 reps)
- A2: Push-ups (to your best effort)

**Superset B** (3 rounds, 90-second rest between rounds)
- B1: Dumbbell deadlift (10–12 reps)
- B2: Bent-over dumbbell row (10–12 reps)

**Core finisher** (3 rounds)
- C1: Plank (hold for as long as possible)

**Cool-down stretch** (5 minutes)

### WHAT'S CHANGED?

Same exercises, same progressive overload principles, but now organised for maximum efficiency. You're doing more work in the same time frame, creating greater metabolic stress and better results. And all while you're at home, too.

Here's how the 40-minute metabolism multiplier works:

1. **Supersets and circuits.** The ultimate efficiency hack. Two exercises back-to-back with zero faff in between. By keeping your heart pumping the entire time your metabolism stays fired

up and you end up burning more calories because you're not sitting around in between sets. Your legs, upper body and your cardiovascular system all get a proper workout in 8 minutes. Example superset that works anywhere:
- 12 goblet squats (using one dumbbell)
- Straight into 10 push-ups (on your knees if needed)
- 20 high knees
- Rest 30–60 seconds, repeat 3 times

2. **Reduced rest periods that maintain metabolic stress.** People think longer rest equals better recovery equals better performance. Sometimes that's true. But when your goal is fat loss and building lean muscle efficiently, shorter rests are your secret weapon. When you cut your rest from 3 minutes down to 90 seconds your muscles don't get to fully recover, so they work harder on the next set. This creates metabolic stress – that burning, fatigued sensation that signals your body to adapt and get stronger. Some may argue that longer rest periods allow you to lift heavier, which is true, but unless you're planning to be the next Dwayne Johnson, you don't need those long rest periods.

At home, this becomes even more powerful because you're not dealing with gym distractions. No one's asking how many sets you have left. No queuing for equipment. You set your timer and you stick to it. If you are doing it in the gym I advise sticking to one piece of equipment and building your supersets around that.

3. **Strategic exercise pairing that allows you to work harder, not longer.** The genius of strategic pairing is that while one muscle group is working, the opposite one is actively recovering.

Pair pushing movements with pulling movements: squats with rows, chest press with back exercises, shoulder press with lat pulldowns. While your chest recovers from push-ups, your back muscles are fresh and ready to work on rows. This means you can perform better on both exercises than if you did them separately.

Even with just a pair of dumbbells in your living room, this becomes incredibly effective. You can do:

- Goblet squats paired with bent-over rows.
- Chest press (lying on the floor) paired with reverse flies.
- Shoulder press paired with bicep curls.

You're getting a full-body workout with minimal equipment, maximum efficiency, and better results than spending 90 minutes wandering around the gym.

4. **Finisher protocols create an afterburn effect lasting hours.** This is where we empty the tank completely. After your main workout, you've got about 3–5 minutes of pure, give it everything you've got intensity.

    These finishers are designed to be brutal but brief. We're talking movements that get your heart rate through the roof and leave you feeling like you've just sprinted up several flights of stairs. The goal isn't to look pretty; it's to create maximum metabolic disruption in minimum time.

    Your three go-to finishers:

    - Tabata burpees: 20 seconds all out, 10 seconds rest, repeat 8 times (4 minutes total).
    - Dumbbell thrusters: As many as you can in 3 minutes straight.
    - Bodyweight circuit: 30 seconds each of jumping jacks, squat jumps, mountain climbers; repeat 3 rounds.

Yes, you might get a bit sweaty. Yes, you might breathe heavily. Yes, you may want to quit 30 seconds in. And yes, if you live in a flat, your downstairs neighbours might wonder what's happening. But it's totally worth it!

The result? You get superior results in less time, with a metabolism that stays elevated long after you've left the gym. This isn't about working harder; it's about working smarter, using science-backed methods to turn your body into a 24-hour fat-burning machine.

> **YOUR PRO TOOLKIT FOR AN EFFECTIVE TRAINING SESSION**
>
> - **Timer aids:** The best tool is a simple timer app on your phone. Pre-programme your work and rest times and press go. The second-best tool is a playlist that is exactly 40 minutes long. When you press play, it's the trigger to train. The end of the playlist is your signal that you're done.
> - **Airplane mode ritual:** Before your first set, put your phone on airplane mode. Make this a non-negotiable. It eliminates the risk of a work email or a social media notification derailing your focus. Remember, this 40 minutes is yours, and yours alone.

## YOUR 'NO EXCUSES' GUIDE

'This all sounds great in a perfect world,' you might be thinking, 'but my world isn't perfect.' Here is your practical, no-excuses playbook for getting a high-density workout done, no matter what life throws at you.

### SCENARIO 1: THE BUSY GYM

You've planned your perfect superset, but the equipment is on opposite sides of a packed gym.

**The pivot:** Ditch the original plan and switch to a 'one-station solution'. Find a quiet corner with a bench and a pair of dumbbells. An example of what your new workout could look like:

**Superset:** Goblet squats and push-ups (with your hands on the bench if needed).

**Superset:** Dumbbell deadlifts and bent-over dumbbell rows.

You can get a phenomenal full-body workout using a small area.

## SCENARIO 2: THE 'I ONLY HAVE A PAIR OF DUMBBELLS AT HOME' PROBLEM

You're working out at home and only have one pair of, say, 8kg dumbbells. They're too light for your squats but too heavy for your shoulder press.

**The pivot:** You will use tempo and rest–pause to manipulate the intensity.

**What is tempo?** Tempo refers to the speed at which you perform each part of an exercise. By slowing down specific phases of the movement, you can make a lighter weight feel much heavier.

**What is rest–pause?** This is when you perform a set until you feel you only have one or two of the repetitions left in you, resting briefly (15–20 seconds), then squeezing out more reps.

### *For your squats, when your weights are too light*

Use a slow, 4-second eccentric.

**What is the 'eccentric'?** The eccentric is the 'lowering' or 'lengthening' part of any exercise – when the muscle is under tension while getting longer. In a squat, this is when you're lowering down into the squat position.

**How to do it:** Take a full 4 seconds to slowly lower yourself down into the squat position, then stand up at normal speed. This increases the time your muscles are under tension, and will make the 8kg feel like 12kg because your muscles are working harder for longer.

***For your shoulder press, when the weight is too heavy***
Use a rest–pause set. Do as many reps as you can (maybe you only get 6), rest for 20 seconds and then immediately try to get another 2 to 3 reps. Repeat one more time. You've just hit your target rep range but in a different way.

## SCENARIO 3: THE 'HOTEL ROOM' BODYWEIGHT BLITZ

You're travelling for work and have no equipment. You have 20 minutes before a dinner meeting.

**The pivot:** Set a timer for 20 minutes and complete as many high-quality rounds as you can of this circuit:

- 10 bodyweight squats
- 8 push-ups (on your knees or using the desk for an incline)
- 12 alternating lunges
- 30-second plank

## SCENARIO 4: THE 'TRAVEL MINI-KIT'

For frequent travellers, investing in a simple 'mini-kit' can be a game-changer. What to pack:

**A resistance band.** Takes up zero space and allows you to do:

- **Rows:** Pull the band towards your chest while holding handles, working your back muscles.

- **Pull-aparts:** Hold the band with both hands and pull it apart at chest level, working your upper back and shoulders.
- **Glute bridge resistance:** Place the band around your thighs and perform glute bridges – the band adds extra resistance to activate your glutes more.

**A skipping rope.** The most efficient and portable piece of cardio equipment on the planet. A 5-minute Tabata with a skipping rope is a brutal but effective finisher.

## TOOLS FOR 'I ONLY HAVE 20 MINUTES' DAYS

These suggested sets are your 'break glass in emergency' options. Follow along on days when you only have 20 minutes available and feel confident you are still making progress despite being strapped for time.

**Please note:** These are advanced techniques for experienced lifters. If you're new to strength training, master the basics first. Stop immediately if you feel any joint pain or sharp discomfort.

### OPTION 1: REST–PAUSE SETS

**What it is:** Do exercise until you feel you have 1–2 good reps left in the tank, then rest for 15–20 seconds, squeeze out a few more reps, rest again, repeat. This lets you use heavier weights than you could for straight 15–20 reps.

**Type of exercise:** Stable exercises like machine press, goblet squats or bicep curls (avoid technical moves like heavy deadlifts).

**How to do it:**
- Choose a weight you can lift for 8–10 reps.
- Perform 8–10 reps until you feel you have 1–2 good reps left in you.

- Rest for 15–20 seconds.
- Squeeze out 3–5 more reps.
- Rest for 15–20 seconds.
- Squeeze out 2–3 final reps.

**Total reps:** 13–18 reps in one extended set
**Time taken:** 2–3 minutes per exercise
**Rest between exercises:** 2–3 minutes

**Benefits gained:** Higher muscle fibre recruitment, greater mechanical tension, and more work done with heavier weights in less time.

## OPTION 2: DROP SETS

**What it is:** Perform this set to where you can't do another move, immediately reduce weight, go to where you can't do another move again. Brutal but effective way to completely exhaust muscle fibres.

**Type of exercise:** Best for isolation exercises with easy weight changes – dumbbell shoulder presses, bicep curls, leg extensions.

**How to do it:**
- Start with your normal working weight.
- Perform 8–12 reps to where you can't do another move.
- Immediately drop weight by 20 to 30 per cent.
- Perform another 6–10 reps to where you can't do another move.
- Drop weight again by 20 to 30 per cent.
- Perform final 4–8 reps to where you can't do another move.

**Total reps:** 18–30 reps in one brutal set
**Time taken:** 2–3 minutes per exercise
**Rest between exercises:** 3–4 minutes (you'll need it!)

**Benefits gained:** Complete muscle exhaustion, massive metabolic stress and maximum muscle fibre recruitment. Use only for your final set of each exercise.

## YOUR NO-NONSENSE FAQs

### 'Can I really get results at home?'
Absolutely. Your muscles only know resistance, not whether that resistance comes from a fancy gym machine or a dumbbell in your living room. Some of the strongest, most confident women I know built their foundation at home with just a set of dumbbells. The gym isn't a graduation requirement – it's just one option. Start where you feel comfortable and confident.

### 'How do I know if I'm pushing too hard or not hard enough?'
Listen to your body's signals. A little muscle stiffness the next day is the sweet spot – it means you challenged yourself appropriately. If you're walking like a cowboy for three days, you overdid it. If you feel nothing at all, you can probably push a bit harder next time. Sharp pain or joint pain is your body saying 'stop immediately' – never push through that.

### 'What if I can't do a full push-up yet?'
Start exactly where you are, not where you think you should be. Use an incline (hands on a bench, couch or wall) or do knee push-ups. Every rep counts. The woman doing perfect knee push-ups is infinitely stronger than the woman sitting on the couch wishing she could do 'real' push-ups. Progress, not perfection.

### 'How long before I see results?'
You'll feel stronger and more confident within 2 weeks – this is real progress, even if it's not visible yet. Others might start noticing physical changes in 4 to 6 weeks, but the most important changes happen in your head first. You start seeing yourself as someone who shows up, someone who follows through, someone who takes care of themselves.

### 'What if I miss a workout? Have I ruined everything?'

Missing one workout is like missing one meal – it literally doesn't matter in the grand scheme of things. The all-or-nothing mindset is what derails people. One missed workout is data, not drama. Just get back to it next time without the guilt spiral.

### 'I feel silly and uncoordinated – is this normal?'

Completely normal. Every expert was once a beginner who felt awkward. Your brain is learning new movement patterns, which takes time. Focus on form over speed or weight. That 'silly' feeling will disappear as you build confidence and competence.

### 'How do I stay motivated when progress feels slow?'

Stop relying on motivation – it's unreliable. Instead, focus on identity. You're not someone trying to get fit; you're someone who moves their body regularly. You're not someone who should exercise; you're someone who does exercise.

---

**FUELLING YOUR SESSIONS**

**Pre-workout (1–2 hours before):** Your goal is easily accessible energy. The golden combo: fast-digesting carbs and a little protein. For example, a banana with a handful of almonds or a rice cake with a spoonful of peanut butter.

**Post-workout (1–2 hours after):** Your goal is replenishment and repair. The golden combo: a significant serving of high-quality protein and some carbs. A full, balanced meal like chicken with sweet potato and veg, or a big protein shake.

So, you've mastered the fundamentals with your weekly workout template from the previous chapter. Now it's time to level up your workout toolbox.

Think of this as your natural progression curve. You started with the basics, learned proper form, and built consistency. Now you're ready to add advanced strategies that will amplify your results without adding more time to your schedule.

### *Your progression journey*

- **Phase 1:** Master the basics with the weekly workout template (you've done this!).
- **Phase 2:** Add intensity techniques for maximum efficiency (that's what we're doing now).
- **Phase 3:** Continue progressing with heavier weights and advanced variations (coming up!).

## YOUR NINTH ACTION PLAN: ENHANCING YOUR TRAINING

**The mindset shift:** Write down one thing your body can do now that it couldn't do when you started this journey. Maybe you sleep better, have more energy, feel stronger. Celebrate that progress – it's evidence that this is working.

**The goal:** To have mastered the fundamentals, and to have moved on to a more economical, effective way to train.

**The task:** Write your enhanced training plan in your logbook. This is your next step up the progression ladder – a more efficient, powerful version of what you've already mastered.

**The practice:** Aim to do strength training 2–3 times per week, focusing on consistent movement that fits your schedule and energy levels.

---

We now have multiple tools in our workout toolbox to get incredible results efficiently. You've evolved your training from basic to advanced. We've built a solid strength foundation – but what about the cardio that you've been told is so essential for fat loss?

In the next chapter, we're going to add the cardio strategies that actually work, and give you permission to skip the stuff that doesn't.

## CHAPTER 10

# CARDIO TO SUPPORT FAT LOSS – AND YOUR SANITY

It's Sunday morning. The room is dark, but you can see the sunlight peeking through the curtains. You've only been awake for a few minutes and you're warm and comfortable in bed when a voice pops into your head, whispering, 'You ate pizza last night. You need to go for a run to burn it off.'

It's the same voice that flooded you with guilt when the calorie counter on your watch showed a lower number after you chose 45 minutes of weights over a spin class for an hour. The one that insists that unless you're drenched in sweat and gasping for air, your workout didn't really happen.

For years, this voice has been your personal drill sergeant, hasn't it? It's made you believe that cardio is penance – payment for the crime of wanting to enjoy food and have a social life.

So, you've done what it demanded. You've dragged yourself to brutal spin classes that left you feeling sick. You've pounded the treadmill until your knees ached. You've pushed through HIIT sessions that made you question your will to live.

And yet ... as we've noted before, you're still here, reading this book, because the cardio approach hasn't worked, has it?

And so this chapter is about (respectfully) telling that drill sergeant to shut up, for good.

We are going to dismantle the myth that punishing cardio is the key to fat loss. I am going to show you why, for a busy, often-stressed woman, your obsession with high-intensity cardio might be the very thing holding you back. We will reframe cardio, moving it from the starring role in your fitness routine to a valuable, strategic supporting actor. You will learn how to use it to support your fat-loss goals, boost your mood and improve your health, without the punishment and without the burnout.

## THE SCIENCE: YOUR BODY'S 'STRESS BUDGET'

To understand the right way to use cardio, we first need to understand one crucial concept: your stress budget.

I want you to imagine that every single day, you wake up with a stress 'budget' of 100 points. Everything you do throughout the day is a withdrawal from this budget.

A bad night's sleep? That's a 20-point withdrawal before you've even opened your eyes.

Skipping breakfast and just having coffee? Minus 10 points. A stressful work meeting? Minus 15 points. An argument with your partner? Minus 20 points. Just the general mental load of running your life? That's another 15 points gone. By 6 p.m., most busy women have already spent their entire 100-point budget, and you are into your stress 'overdraft'.

Now, let's look at exercise. All exercise is a physical stressor – that's how it creates change. But different types of exercise make very different withdrawals from your budget. A restorative,

30-minute walk in nature might only be a 5-point withdrawal. It might even feel like a deposit. A 45-minute, focused strength-training session is a strategic, worthwhile 25-point withdrawal. A brutal, 45-minute, all-out HIIT class? For a body that is already in its stress overdraft, that is a massive 50-point withdrawal.

When you consistently overdraw from your stress budget, your body does what any financial manager might do: it panics. It perceives this as a state of chronic crisis. It floods your system with cortisol, which, as we know, signals to your body to store belly fat, break down precious muscle and disrupt your sleep.

The reason so many women burn out is that they are trying to pay for their fat loss with a currency they simply don't have. They are trying to make huge, 50-point cardio training withdrawals from an already overdrawn account, pushing themselves ever deeper into hormonal debt. Our goal is to be smart investors in our stress budget. We want to choose the forms of cardio that give us the biggest health and fat-loss return for the smallest possible withdrawal.

### YOUR TWO NEW CARDIO TOOLS: THE TORTOISE AND THE HARE

There are two main types of cardio: high-intensity interval training, and low-intensity steady state.

For years, you've been told that HIIT is the hare, the hero. I'm here to tell you that for most of us, most of the time, the more tortoise-like LISS is the real winner.

#### 1. LISS (low-intensity steady state): the tortoise

This is any movement where you could hold a conversation without gasping. Think brisk walking (especially uphill), easy cycling or a gentle session on the cross-trainer.

**Why it works:** LISS primarily burns fat for fuel. It supports your nervous system rather than overwhelming it. It improves blood flow, helps with recovery and makes you feel better rather than completely knackered.

**When to use it:** This should be your bread and butter. Perfect for off-days from strength training; as a warm-up; or any time you want to move your body without adding stress to your system.

### 2. HIIT (high-intensity interval training): the hare

Short, all-out bursts followed by rest periods. Think sprints, burpees or those assault bike sessions that make you question your life choices.

**Why it works:** HIIT is incredibly effective for improving fitness and creating an 'afterburn' effect in minimal time. It's like a shot of espresso for your metabolism. The catch is it's also like drinking ten shots of espresso when you're already wired. Powerful, but it needs to be used strategically.

**When to use it:** Sparingly. Think of HIIT as an expensive perfume – a little goes a long way. For most women, once or twice a week maximum, preferably as a short finisher after strength training.

You need to stop trying to be the hare every day. Embrace your inner tortoise. Slow, steady and consistent wins the fat-loss race.

# THE 'MINIMAL EFFECTIVE DOSE' PRESCRIPTION

The idea of favouring gentle LISS over intense HIIT can be a hard pill to swallow, especially for high-achievers. Your brain is wired to think that if a little bit of something is good, then more must be better. If a 10-minute HIIT session is effective, then a 45-minute one must be a fat-loss miracle, right?

Wrong. This is where we need to introduce the powerful concept of the minimal effective dose (MED).

Think of it like a medical prescription. If you have a headache and your doctor tells you to take two paracetamol tablets, you take two. You don't swallow the entire box thinking it will cure your headache faster or more effectively. You understand that taking more than the prescribed dose won't lead to better results; it will lead to a toxic overdose and a new set of problems.

HIIT is a powerful medicine for your metabolism. It is a potent, acute stressor that can trigger a fantastic adaptive response. But your prescription should be a small one. For most women, the minimal effective dose of HIIT is 5 to 10 minutes, once or, at most, twice a week. Taking more than this doesn't lead to better results. It leads to the negative side effects of an overdose: chronically elevated cortisol, systemic inflammation, ravenous hunger, joint pain and burnout.

Your new, smarter approach is to stop thinking like a maximalist and start thinking like a skilled physician. You will use the lowest dose necessary to get the desired effect. This reframes 'doing less' not as a compromise or a sign of laziness, but as a smarter, more precise and ultimately more effective strategy.

### EMMA'S STORY

Emma was a classic 'hare'. A 28-year-old account director, she was convinced that her twice-weekly, vomit-inducing HIIT classes were the key to her fat-loss goals. She would go into the class, smash herself for 45 minutes and feel a sense of virtuous accomplishment. But she was also constantly exhausted, her progress had stalled and she found that after her HIIT class, she was so ravenously hungry that she would often 'reward' herself with a huge, carb-heavy meal that would undo all her hard work. She came to me frustrated. 'I'm working as hard as I possibly can in those classes,' she said. 'Why isn't it working?'

I explained the stress budget to her. Her high-stress job and busy social life meant she was already running on empty. Her intense HIIT classes were not a solution; they were flammable, pouring more cortisol onto her already raging stress fire.

Her new plan felt ridiculously easy to her at first. We kept her three weekly strength sessions, but we replaced her two brutal HIIT classes with two 40-minute, brisk incline walks on the treadmill while she listened to a podcast.

She was sceptical. 'But I'm barely even sweating!' she said after the first week. But by week three, the changes were undeniable. 'I don't get it,' she messaged me. 'My sleep is better. I'm not getting that insane post-workout hunger anymore. And I feel ... calmer. And my waist feels smaller.'

Emma didn't need to work harder. She needed to work smarter. By swapping her high-stress cardio for low-stress cardio, she finally gave her body a chance to get out of survival mode, lower its cortisol and start burning fat effectively.

## A PRACTICAL GUIDE TO YOUR CARDIO TOOLS

'Okay,' you're thinking. 'I get LISS and HIIT. But what does that look like in the gym or at home? What machines should I use? How fast should I go?'

Let's get practical.

## YOUR LISS TOOLKIT

The goal for LISS is to keep your heart rate in a steady, moderate zone. The simplest way to measure this is the 'talk test': you should be able to hold a conversation without gasping for breath whilst exercising.

### *The gold standard*
**Incline walking:** In my opinion, this is the most effective and accessible form of LISS. It's low-impact, great for your posture and brilliant for fat burning.

- On a treadmill: aim for a speed of 3.5 to 4.5 mph and an incline of 8 to 12 per cent for 30 to 45 minutes.
- Outside: Find hills, or stride out on flat ground for 30 to 45 minutes.

**The gym classics:** Cross-trainer or stationary bike. Both are fantastic, low-impact options.

- Find a resistance level that feels like a 6/10 effort. You should feel you're working, but you could sustain it for 45 minutes.

## YOUR HIIT TOOLKIT

The goal for HIIT is to go all-out, to a 9/10 or 10/10 level of effort, during your work intervals.

### *The gold standard*
**The 30/30 assault bike or spin bike finisher**
**The protocol:** Go all-out for 30 seconds. Then, pedal slowly for 30 seconds of active recovery. Repeat 10 times. It's a brutal but brilliant 10-minute finisher.

### The 10-minute treadmill sprint finisher

**The protocol:** Sprint for 20 seconds at a challenging speed. Then, step your feet onto the sides of the treadmill and rest for 40 seconds. Repeat 10 times.

### The bodyweight Tabata finisher

**The protocol:** Choose one explosive bodyweight move (like burpees or jumping squats). Go all-out for 20 seconds. Rest for 10 seconds. Repeat 8 times. A classic 4-minute finisher you can do anywhere.

## THE SYSTEM: WEAVING CARDIO INTO YOUR WEEK

### RULE 1

Strength first, always. As we know, your strength-training sessions are your non-negotiable 'metabolic pension' deposits: every strength-training session builds muscle tissue that works for you 24/7. Unlike cardio that burns calories only while you're doing it, the muscle you build keeps burning energy even while you sleep. This is why consistent strength training is one of the most effective long-term strategies for metabolic health. Your cardio should just be a supporting player. If you're doing both on the same day, always do your strength workout first, when you are fresh, and finish with your cardio.

### RULE 2

Aim for 8,000 to 10,000 steps daily as your foundation. But here's the thing – if you're currently averaging 2,000 steps, don't jump straight to 10,000. That's a recipe for burnout. Instead, follow the 'Add 2,000 and stabilise' rule: if you're averaging 2,000 steps, aim for 4,000 for two weeks. Once that feels automatic, bump it up to 6,000 for another two weeks. Then work towards your

8,000 target. This is about working smart. Remember, sustainable changes stick. Dramatic changes don't.

## RULE 3

Make LISS your default. Aim for one to three sessions of 30 to 45 minutes LISS cardio per week. The best time to do this is on your 'off days' from strength training. This is your active recovery.

## RULE 4

Use HIIT as a finisher. If you enjoy the intensity of HIIT, use it as a strategic, 5- to 10-minute finisher at the end of one or two of your strength workouts per week. This gives you the metabolic bang for your buck without the full-body burnout.

# COMMON MISTAKES THAT CAN SABOTAGE YOUR CARDIO

**Mistake:** Doing LISS too intensely – you got on the cross-trainer for your 'gentle' session but couldn't resist cranking up the resistance until you're breathing heavily.

**The fix:** You've accidentally turned your LISS into moderate-intensity cardio. This can be more draining than it is restorative. Stick to the talk test. If you can't hold a conversation, you're going too hard. Lower the intensity.

**Mistake:** Doing HIIT on an empty stomach to 'burn more fat'.

**The fix:** This is a recipe for muscle breakdown and a huge cortisol spike. HIIT is a high-intensity activity that requires glucose for fuel. Always do it in a well-fed state (i.e. not first thing in the morning before breakfast).

**Mistake:** Letting your step count drop to zero on strength days.

**The fix:** Your daily step count is your foundation. The 8,000- to 10,000-step goal applies *every* day. Your strength workout is the bonus, not the replacement for your general daily movement.

> ### MAKE IT STICK: BUILDING THE HABIT OF MOVEMENT
>
> **The tiny habit:** The single most powerful habit you can embed is a 10-minute walk after your evening meal. It's non-negotiable. It aids digestion, helps to manage your blood sugar and creates a clear separation from your day.
>
> **The environment tweak:** Put your trainers by the sofa to remind you before sitting down. This visual cue removes the friction of having to 'get ready' and makes the decision to go for a walk almost automatic.
>
> **The if–then plan:** Create a plan for your biggest excuse. '*If* it's raining and I can't do my evening walk, *then* I will spend 15 minutes walking up and down in my house while listening to a podcast or relaxing music.'

# THE REAL-WORLD GUIDE: INCREASING YOUR STEPS WITH 'HABIT STACKING'

If you're thinking: 'Finding time for multiple strength workouts *and* one to three cardio sessions per week while hitting my steps sounds like a lot,' then I encourage you to stop thinking in terms of hour-long 'sessions', and start thinking in terms of 'stacking' movement into your existing day. Nobody explains that your step count matters more than any structured cardio session. Getting 8,000 to 10,000 steps by walking is like having a gentle, fat-burning engine running all day. It doesn't stress your system, it improves your mood and it's completely free.

### Habit-stacking wins to boost your steps

- **The commute stack:** Get off the bus or train one stop early and walk the rest of the way.
- **The lunchbreak add on:** After you eat your lunch, immediately go for a 15-minute brisk walk.
- **The walking phone call:** Have a rule that any non-video work call is taken while pacing around your office or your living room.
- **The end of day decompress:** The moment you finish work, put on your trainers and walk around the block for 10 minutes before you start your evening. This creates a powerful mental and physical separation from your workday.
- **The post-dinner ritual:** After your evening meal, take a 10-minute walk around the block. This isn't just about steps – it helps with digestion, blood sugar control, and creates a natural transition into your evening wind-down routine. Make it non-negotiable.

These small, stacked habits are often far more effective and sustainable than trying to find a whole new 45-minute slot in your diary.

## DON'T HIIT YOUR HORMONES

We'll look more at hormones in the next chapter, but for now we need to be clear that our menstrual cycle can definitely affect your ability to work out.

**First half of your cycle (power phase):** This is a great time to incorporate those short, sharp HIIT finishers (5 to 10 minutes after your strength sessions). Your body is more resilient to stress at this time.

**Second half of your cycle (luteal phase):** As you approach your period, your body is under more physiological stress. Have you ever tried to force yourself through a high-intensity workout the week before your period and felt like you were moving through mud? You're not being lazy or weak; you are pushing against your own physiology.

During your luteal phase, your joints can be laxer, and your body is more sensitive to the stress hormone, cortisol. Pushing through a brutal workout can actually be counterproductive, jacking up cortisol even more, which can worsen PMS, disrupt sleep and increase cravings.

This is the time to favour gentle LISS.

**The smart deload approach:** A 'deload' isn't skipping your workout; it's being smart. It's choosing a form of movement that nourishes your body in its current state instead of depleting it. Instead of the HIIT session, swap for an extra 20-minute walk. Instead of trying to hit a personal best on your deadlift, do a lighter-weight session with more reps, or switch to a yoga class.

### DIFFERENT LIFESTYLES, DIFFERENT TWEAKS

- **Shift workers:** Your body clock is already under immense stress. Punishing HIIT sessions are not a good idea. Your focus should be on gentle, restorative movement. Try to get some LISS cardio in after you wake up (during your 'morning'), ideally in natural daylight if possible, to help regulate your circadian rhythm.

- **New mums:** Your stress budget is already maxed out with sleep deprivation, hormonal changes and the mental load of caring for a baby. Gentle walks with the pram are perfect LISS – you're getting movement, fresh air and potentially some mental space. Save HIIT until you're sleeping more consistently and feeling stronger.

- **Working mums:** You're juggling work stress with family demands. Your cardio should feel like a break, not another stressor. Morning walks before the house wakes up or evening walks after bedtime can be both exercise and much-needed mental reset time. Choose LISS over HIIT most days.

- **High-stress-job workers:** If your job is chronically stressful (think healthcare workers, teachers, emergency services), your stress bucket is already overflowing. Gentle, rhythmic movement like walking or cycling helps lower cortisol rather than adding to it. Use exercise as stress relief, not stress creation.

## CARDIO ON THE GO: THE TRAVEL AND MINIMAL KIT GUIDE

'How do I keep this up when I'm travelling and don't have access to a gym?' The answer is to keep it simple and focus on the basics.

### YOUR LISS WORKOUT

**The tool:** Your trainers.

**The protocol:** The best way to get your LISS cardio done when you're in a new city is to walk. Ditch the taxi or the train for one journey a day and explore on foot. Aim to add an extra 5,000 steps on top of your daily count.

## YOUR HIIT WORKOUT

**The tool:** Your skipping rope.

**The protocol:** Find a small space with enough room to swing a rope – your hotel room (if the ceilings are high enough), a quiet hallway, courtyard or outdoor area. Perform a 5-minute Tabata: 20 seconds of fast skipping, 10 seconds of rest. Repeat 10 times. This is a phenomenal way to get a quick metabolic boost and shake off travel fatigue.

## YOUR TENTH ACTION PLAN: EMBRACE THE TORTOISE

**The mindset shift:** Next time you take a phone call, walk. Whether it's your mum, your friend, or a work call – put your feet in motion. This transforms 'dead time' into movement time.

**The goal:** To prove to yourself that you can seamlessly integrate more low-stress movement into your life without it feeling like a chore.

### PART 1: THE STEP AUDIT – THIS WEEK'S MISSION

**The task:** For the next seven days, your only goal is to become aware of your current baseline for your steps.

**The action:** Use your phone or watch to track your daily step count, without trying to change anything. At the end of the week, find your daily average. This is your starting point. Remember: no judgment, just data.

### PART 2: BUILD YOUR STEP LADDER

**The task:** Looking at the habit-stacking list on page 203, choose one of the strategies that feels easiest to implement.

**The action:** For the next week, commit to doing just that one thing every day. Maybe it's the 10-minute walk after work, or the walking phone calls.

Congratulations. You have learned the final secret of smart training. You have the tools to build a strong, metabolically active body, and you have a plan to support it with intelligent, stress-friendly cardio. You have the complete engine.

Now, we need to make sure that engine can run smoothly, even on the messiest, most chaotic days. In the next chapter, we are going to build your resilience plan for when life – invariably – gets in the way.

## CHAPTER 11
# YOUR PSYCHOLOGICAL FIRST-AID KIT FOR CHALLENGING DAYS

It happens in an instant: one moment, you're in control of your day; the next, a switch has been flipped. It's not a thought, it's a physical force – a magnetic pull towards the kitchen, a sudden and total obsession with the idea of something sweet, salty or carb-related. Your rational brain, the one looking after all your goals and best intentions, seems to vanish. In its place is a single, powerful, non-negotiable directive: *I need it now.*

This is not the loud, critical voice of the drill sergeant we silenced in the earlier chapter. This is something else entirely. It's a seductive, urgent whisper that promises a single, beautiful thing: *relief.* It promises a momentary escape from the stress of your inbox, a soft landing after a chaotic day with the kids, a comforting buffer against boredom or loneliness. It promises that for the next few minutes, the pressure will lift. And in that moment, the promise feels more appealing than anything else in the world.

This intense, overwhelming urge is not a character flaw. It is a biological SOS signal. It's a flare fired by an overwhelmed nervous system, a desperate attempt by your brain to find the fastest path to safety and comfort. For years, the only tool you've had for this job is food. It's fast, it's reliable and it works – but only temporarily.

This chapter will give you a better toolkit. A more sophisticated one. We are going to move beyond the shame and the mystery around cravings to build a psychological first-aid kit. This is not about white-knuckling your way through temptation. This is about learning to become a calm, skilled first responder to your own emotional and biological needs. You will learn to diagnose what your body is asking for and apply the right treatment, so that you can navigate these moments with confidence, compassion and a profound sense of power.

This is where you stop being hijacked and start being the pilot.

## TOOL 1: THE CRAVING DECISION SEQUENCE

As we've already seen, when a sudden, intense craving hijacks your brain, your mind presents you with only two options: fight a miserable, willpower battle you'll probably lose, or give in completely and deal with the guilt later.

This tool offers you a powerful third path. We're not going to fight the craving, and we're not going to surrender to it. We are going to get *curious* about it. Our mantra for this process is simple: diagnose, don't deny.

Think of it as the calm, diagnostic protocol you use when a warning light flashes on your car's dashboard. You don't panic or ignore it; you pull over and figure out what the signal means. You can do the same for cravings.

Using the series of simple questions below, you can check in with your body to find out what it truly needs.

### *'Am I thirsty?'*

Before you take a single step towards the kitchen, your first action is to drink one full glass of water. This isn't a trick to fill you up: it's your first and most important diagnostic test. The part of your brain that manages thirst and hunger can easily get its wires crossed, especially when you're stressed or busy. After you've finished the glass, pause for five full minutes. Set a timer. You might feel the urge to just rush to the next step, but this pause is where the magic happens. It's the space where your body can reset its signals. You will be astonished at how often the roaring fire of a craving is extinguished by a simple glass of water, once you give it a moment to work.

### *'Am I actually hungry?'*

If the signal is still there after your five-minute pause, it's time for the next question. A frantic craving is often a direct symptom of unstable blood sugar. Your body is screaming for quick energy. Instead of reaching for the 'kindling' (a biscuit) that will burn out in minutes and leave you crashing again, your job is to provide a 'solid log' to create steady, enduring energy. Give your body a protein anchor.

Don't have a boiled egg? No problem. This can be a handful of nuts, two spoonfuls of cottage cheese or Greek yogurt from the fridge, a slice of turkey or even a glass of milk. The goal is a quick hit of protein to stabilise your system. This single act is incredibly empowering, as it proves the craving wasn't for a biscuit, it was for *stability*.

### *'Is this feeling or is this fact?'*

If you're hydrated, have eaten protein and the craving still whispers to you, you've just gathered invaluable data. You can now be confident that this is an emotional wave, not a physical need. This is where the 15-minute rule comes in.

Set a timer and tell yourself, with genuine permission: 'I can eat it in 15 minutes if I still want it.' Then immediately use that time to apply one of our stress scripts (coming up on page 215). This 15-minute window isn't about enduring torture – it's an active treatment period.

You're giving the emotional wave time to pass while addressing its root cause.

### 'Do I still want this?'

When the timer sounds, check in. With luck that frantic, desperate feeling is gone. The wave has passed. You've arrived at a place of calm authority.

But what if you still want it? Here's the most important part: even if you decide to eat the biscuit, you have already won. You broke the automatic, unconscious loop. You went from panicked reaction to conscious, deliberate decision. That's a monumental victory.

If you choose to eat it, you do so on your terms – mindfully, deliberately and without a shred of guilt, because you've proved you're the one in charge.

This four-step process does more than manage a craving. It fundamentally rebuilds the trust between you and your body. Every time you run this diagnostic, you're rewriting years of programming and proving to yourself that you're not at the mercy of your urges. You can ask the questions and deliver the answers, too.

Our philosophy is this: Ride the wave, don't fight the tide.

This is the art of 'urge surfing'.

## TOOL 2: HOW TO 'URGE SURF' WITH CONFIDENCE

At first, doing all this will feel strange and uncomfortable. That's okay. It's a new skill. The first few times you try, your only goal is to stay on the surfboard, and not get knocked off. Try this:

- **Name it:** Acknowledge what's happening without being unkind to yourself. Say, 'Right, this is a craving. It's a big wave of urgency.' Naming it separates you from the feeling. You're not the craving; you're the one watching the craving.
- **Notice where you feel it:** Where is this urge sitting in your body? A hollow feeling in your stomach? Tension in your jaw? Restless hands? Get curious about it. Just notice these physical feelings without letting them to disappear. When you focus on the sensation, you'll stop listening to the story the craving is telling you ('I absolutely must have chocolate right now or I'll die!').
- **Breathe into it:** Imagine you can breathe right into that part of your body. Breathe into the tension, the restlessness, the hollow feeling. This is the difference between fighting and observing. Fighting is tensing up against the wave. Observing is staying relaxed on the board, letting the energy move through you.

### But won't focusing on it make it stronger?

This is the mental part of urge surfing. The urge gets its power from your resistance to it. When you fight it, you fuel it. When you calmly and curiously observe it, you rob it of any power. You are effectively unplugging it from its energy source. You are watching the wave, not becoming the wave.

### The science of rewiring your brain

It's amazing what is going in your head during these 15 minutes. You're rewiring your brain. Every time you successfully surf an urge, you're weakening that old automatic pathway: *Feel thing* → *Eat thing* → *Feel better then worse.* You are now building a new, stronger one: *Feel thing* → *Watch thing* → *Handle it.*

You're proving to your brain that it doesn't need the food to get through the uncomfortable feeling. You're teaching it that it can manage the wave on its own. This isn't just a coping trick – you're upgrading your brain.

### What if 15 minutes feels impossible?

Start with five. If five minutes feels like a lifetime, start with two. The goal is not to be a perfect surfer on day one. The goal is to simply get on the board. Each time you practise – for one minute or fifteen – you are strengthening mental muscle and proving to yourself that you are not at the mercy of the tide.

This is where your stress scripts will come in handy – they're like your compass, helping you navigate through the wave with purpose instead of just hanging on for dear life.

## TOOL 3: STRESS SCRIPTS

You've completed your decision sequence, been through the steps and urge-surfed through your 15-minute window. This has helped to work out what's going on in your brain.

Your stress scripts come next – these are the formulas you can apply to your brain to provide relief.

A truly effective stress script isn't just a random distraction. It's built on three core principles. Think of it as your 'three Rs formula' for creating comfort.

- **REPLACE:** It must replace the physical action of eating with another simple, physical action.

- **REGULATE:** It must actively regulate your nervous system (calming you down or gently stimulating you).
- **REWARD:** It must provide a genuine sense of relief, accomplishment or pleasure – an emotional payoff.

Let me show you how this works in real life.

## 1. FOR 'MY BRAIN WON'T SHUT UP' OVERWHELM, YOU NEED CALM

**The old script:** Mindless eating to numb the mental noise.

**Action:** Go to your kitchen and make a cup of herbal tea (peppermint or chamomile work well). The ritual is the entire process: filling the kettle, waiting for it to boil, watching the steam, holding the warm mug in your hands. For three minutes, your only job is to focus on the sensory experience – the warmth, the smell, the taste.

**The three Rs breakdown:** This sequence replaces eating with drinking. It regulates your nervous system through warmth and calming aromas. It rewards you with a genuine moment of peace and a break from any screens. It pulls you out of your racing thoughts and plants you firmly in the present moment.

## 2. FOR 'I'M COMPLETELY KNACKERED' EXHAUSTION, YOU NEED COMFORT

**The old script:** A hit of sugar as a 'reward' for surviving the day.

**Action:** Go to your bedroom or a comfortable chair. Do you have a favourite soft blanket or a soft sweater? Wrap yourself in it. Put on a pair of warm socks. Apply a pleasant-smelling lip balm or hand lotion. For five minutes, just sit or lie down in your comfort cocoon and breathe.

**The three Rs breakdown:** This sequence replaces eating with touch and warmth. It regulates your system through cosiness and gentle pressure (which is deeply calming). It rewards you with a feeling of safety and genuine self-care that a chocolate bar can never provide.

### 3. FOR 'I'M SO BORED I COULD SCREAM' RESTLESSNESS, YOU NEED ENGAGEMENT

**The old script:** Grazing on snacks to fill the void and provide stimulation.

**Action:** Look around you. Is there a tiny, five-minute task that would make 'tomorrow-you' feel amazing? It could be wiping down the kitchen counters, putting one load of laundry in the machine, replying to that one nagging text or tidying the pile of shoes by the door. Set a timer for five minutes and attack that one task.

**The three Rs breakdown:** This sequence is designed to give your brain the hit of dopamine it seeks from engagement, but in a productive way. It replaces mindless eating with mindful action. It regulates your restlessness by giving it a focus point. It rewards you with a powerful hit of accomplishment and a calmer environment, which is far more satisfying than the quick pleasure of a snack.

## WHY HORMONES MATTER MORE THAN WILLPOWER

As we've seen, your hormones are constantly shifting throughout the month, responding to stress, food choices, exercise and sleep patterns. One week you might feel like you could conquer the world, the next you're face-first in a bag of crisps wondering what happened to your motivation.

### *The main players you need to know about*

- **Insulin** – Your blood sugar manager (goes crazy when you eat refined carbs on an empty stomach).
- **Cortisol** – Your stress hormone (brilliant in small doses, destructive when constantly elevated).
- **Oestrogen and progesterone** – Your cycle hormones (create a monthly rollercoaster of energy, mood, and cravings).
- **Leptin and ghrelin** – Your hunger and fullness signals (get scrambled by poor sleep and stress).
- **Thyroid hormones** – Your metabolic accelerator (slows down when you're chronically stressed or under-eating).

The good news? Once you understand how these work together, you can start working with them instead of against them. No more wondering why you felt brilliant last week but terrible this week. No more blaming yourself for cravings that are actually hormonally driven. Remember: there's nothing wrong with you. Your body is designed to respond to hormonal signals. When you learn to read these signals and respond appropriately, everything becomes easier.

## HORMONE HACKS FOR TOUGH DAYS

If you have PCOS or your hormones are just generally having a bit of a rave (your period might show up twice in one month and then ghost you for the next three), trying to map that onto a neat 28-day cycle chart feels like trying to force a cat into a party dress. It's pointless, stressful and someone's going to get scratched.

For years, I felt like my body was a glitch. Broken. But here's the secret I had to learn the hard way: your period (or lack thereof) is not the problem. That's the outcome. When you don't have a predictable cycle, you don't track the *outcome* (your period); you track the *signals*. Instead, we become skilful detectives. We start looking for clues and gathering gossip.

Here are the clues you're looking for. Forget the period apps for a minute. All you need is the notes app on your phone, or a diary.

## DETECTIVE CLUE SHEET

Every day, jot down a few notes on these four things. It takes less than two minutes.

### *1. Your energy score (out of 10)*

This is your body's battery level. Is it fully charged, or are you running on fumes? Be brutally honest. 1/10 is: 'I can't even be bothered to find the TV remote' or 'I've made a permanent dent in the sofa.' 10/10 is: 'I could conquer a small country before lunch' or 'I've already cleaned the house, answered all my emails, and am considering taking up a new language.'

Just jot down the number. After a while, you'll see a pattern. Maybe you have two weeks of high energy followed by a week-long crash. That's your pattern.

### *2. Your mood and vibe*

Hormones are the puppet masters of our moods. So, what's the general vibe today?

- **Are you feeling generally chill and capable?** Like you can handle whatever life throws at you?
- **Are you feeling anxious or weepy?** Like a sad song in an advert could send you over the edge?
- **Are you feeling snappy and irritable?** Do you want to bite someone's head off for breathing too loudly?

Just one word is fine: 'Chilled,' 'Anxious,' 'Rage-y.' It's all good data.

### 3. The cravings report

Your appetite is a direct message from your hormones and your blood sugar.

- **Is your body politely asking for nourishing food?** Are you feeling fairly stable and in control around food?
- **Is it a screaming, hormonal monster?** Is it demanding that you drive to a 24-hour garage for a family-sized bag of crisps and a chocolate bar the size of your head?

Note it down: 'Stable hunger' vs 'Ravenous monster.' You'll start to see that your 'ravenous monster' days often line up with your low-energy, rage-y days. See? Detective work.

### 4. Your skin's gossip column

My skin was always the biggest snitch. It told the entire world what was going on inside me. What is your skin telling you?

- **Is it calm and clear?**
- **Is it oily?**
- **Has a new, angry friend decided to move in on your chin?**

Just a quick note: 'Skin calm' or 'New chin monster'.
    Once you've got the hang of the basics, you can add two more clues that are absolute game-changers for hormonal health.

### 5. The sleep report

Was your sleep amazing, or was it horrific? Did you fall asleep easily but wake up at 3 a.m. to make endless to-do lists in your head? Sleep quality is a direct reflection of your stress hormones. Note: 'Slept like the dead' or 'Woke up 5 times'.

### 6. The poo report

Yes, we're going there. Your poo is a daily report card from your gut, and your gut health is everything when it comes to hormones. Is everything moving along nicely, or is it a bit of a traffic jam? You don't need to write a novel about it. Note: 'Happy gut' or 'Struggling'.

After a couple of weeks of this, you'll have a treasure trove of information. You can scroll back and see it plain as day: 'Huh! Look at that. The first week of the month, I had 8/10 energy, my mood was great and my skin was calm. Then, around day 14, everything shifted – my energy stayed high but I craved more carbs. By day 21, my energy crashed to a 4/10, I wanted to cry at everything and I was desperate for carbs for three days straight. Then around day 26, I felt more balanced again, just a bit more tired than usual.'

And here's the thing – your cycle might be 25 days, 32 days or completely irregular. The key is learning YOUR pattern.

## NAVIGATING EXERCISE DURING PERIMENOPAUSE AND MENOPAUSE

If you're in your 40s or 50s and finding that your usual exercise routine suddenly feels harder, you're not imagining things. Hormonal shifts during perimenopause and menopause directly impact how your body handles stress and recovers from workouts.

Your stress budget becomes more unpredictable. Fluctuating hormones can leave you energetic one day and drained the next. This isn't a sign you're 'getting old' – it's your body navigating a major transition that requires a more flexible approach to exercise.

## The key adjustments

- **Listen to your body daily:** Some days you'll feel strong enough for intense training; others you'll need gentle movement. Both are equally valuable.
- **Prioritise strength training:** As oestrogen declines, you lose muscle faster. Consistent strength sessions are your insurance policy against bone loss and metabolic slowdown.
- **Work with your energy, not against it:** Poor sleep night? Swap HIIT for a walk. Your recovery time may be longer now – that's wisdom, not weakness.
- **Focus on how you feel:** The scale might fluctuate more due to hormonal changes, but your strength, energy and confidence are better progress measures.

This isn't about accepting less – it's about working smarter with your changing physiology to stay strong for the decades ahead.

# WHEN THE THREE RS NEED BACKUP: 10 RED FLAGS TO SEE YOUR GP

Okay, let's have a very important, very real chat. We've talked a lot in this book about becoming the expert on your own body, and that is your superpower. But part of being a good expert is knowing when to bring in a consultant. Your GP is that person.

For too long, women have been patted on the head and told that their pain, their exhaustion and their weird symptoms are 'just stress', 'part of being a woman', or something that can be fixed if they just 'lose a bit of weight'.

We are done with that.

The following list is your permission slip. It's your guide to knowing when your symptoms have crossed the line from 'annoying hormonal stuff' into 'this needs a proper medical look'.

If any of this sounds like you, your job is not to panic. Your job is to calmly pick up the phone and make an appointment.

1. **Your periods have gone nuclear:** We're not talking about your standard day-one cramps. We're talking about pain that painkillers can't touch, that makes you cancel plans, or bleeding so heavy you're soaking through a super tampon or pad every hour or two. This is not normal, and you do not have to 'just put up with it'.
2. **Your period has gone on holiday and forgotten to send a postcard:** If you've missed three or more periods in a row (and you're not pregnant), your body is sending up a major flare. It's a sign that something is significant enough to shut down your reproductive system, and it needs investigating.
3. **There's bleeding when there shouldn't be:** This means spotting between your periods, or bleeding after sex. It might be nothing to worry about, but it's one of those things that absolutely must be checked out by a doctor. No exceptions.
4. **Your PMS has gone from 'a bit grumpy' to 'full-blown rage monster':** If your mood swings in the week before your period are so severe that they are genuinely wrecking your relationships, your work or your sanity, you could have PMDD (premenstrual dysphoric disorder). This is a real, treatable medical condition, not just 'bad PMS'.
5. **You're exhausted at a soul-deep level:** This isn't just 'I'm a bit tired.' This is bone-crushing fatigue where you could sleep for 10 hours and still wake up feeling like you've been run over. It can be a sign of thyroid issues, severe iron deficiency or other things that need a blood test to uncover.
6. **You're fighting a losing battle with new hair growth:** If you're noticing new, dark, coarse hairs growing on your face, chest or

back, or if the hair on your head is noticeably thinning, these can be hallmark signs of the hormonal imbalances seen in PCOS, which a doctor can help you with.
7. **Sex is painful:** It's that simple. Sex should not be painful. If it is, it can be a sign of things like endometriosis, fibroids or pelvic floor issues. A good doctor will take this seriously.
8. **You've had a sudden, weird weight change:** If you've gained or lost a significant amount of weight without any major changes to your diet or exercise routine, it's worth a conversation. Your thyroid or other hormones could be playing up.
9. **Perimenopause symptoms are ruining your life:** If hot flashes, night sweats, brain fog or anxiety are so bad they're affecting your ability to sleep, work or just feel like a normal human being, please go and talk to your doctor. There are so many options now, including modern HRT, that can give you your life back. You do not have to suffer in silence.
10. **Something just feels *wrong*:** This is the most important one of all. You live in your body. You know what feels normal for you. If you have a nagging feeling that something isn't right, even if you can't quite put your finger on it, that is reason enough to make an appointment. Trust your gut.

When you go to that appointment, walk in with notes you've been taking. Show the GP your patterns. Be calm, be clear and don't let anyone fob you off. You are not a hypochondriac. You are an expert in your own experience, and you deserve a partner in your health.

# YOUR ELEVENTH ACTION PLAN: RECOGNISE THE SIGNS

**The mindset shift:** Recognise that overwhelm, exhaustion, hormones or boredom can be your biggest downfalls, and learn to spot them for what they are.

**The goal:** To create your own three Rs stress scripts that work with your hormonal patterns and are tailored specifically to you.

**The task:** Grab a piece of paper or open the notes app on your phone. Using the three Rs formula, design your own go-to stress script. Think about your hormonal patterns you've been tracking – when do you typically feel most vulnerable to stress eating? Is it during your pre-menstrual phase when progesterone drops and you're craving carbs? During ovulation when your energy dips? Or maybe when you're sleep-deprived and your hunger hormones are going haywire? What physical action can you replace stress eating with? How will it regulate your nervous system? What is the genuine reward you'll feel? Be specific and consider how this might need to change depending on where you are in your cycle.

**The practice:** Don't worry about getting it perfect. Your first script is a draft. The practice is to try it out during your next challenging moment – whether that's hormone-driven cravings, stress from work, or just general overwhelm. If it works, brilliant. If it doesn't, you haven't failed – you've collected data. You can tweak the script until it becomes the perfect, custom-fit relief your body was asking for all along, whether you're dealing with PMS munchies or stress-induced carb cravings.

This is not about following rules; it's about becoming your own expert on what your body and hormones need.

# MILESTONE 2: THE 'MESSY MIDDLE' CHALLENGE

Let's pause. We're 11 chapters in. You've survived the initial phase. You're getting the hang of the food and training. But you've probably hit some turbulence along the way. Perhaps you've experienced a craving that felt like a hijacking? Or you've heard mean whispers from your inner critic after a day where it all felt too hard.

This is normal. This is the messy middle.

This is the part of the journey where the real dragons show up. The dragons aren't the food on your plate; they are the feelings in your head. Self-doubt creeps in, or subtle social pressure makes you want to abandon all your new habits.

The next seven days will be your training ground for learning how to *dance* with these dragons. We're not trying to slay them; we're learning their moves so they no longer have power over us. We are going to take your new skills out into the wild, away from the comfort of your own routine. The aim is not to reach perfection but to prove your resilience. Welcome to the messy middle challenge.

## YOUR 7-DAY MISSION: THE POWER PRACTICE

We are going on a scavenger hunt. Your mission is to find opportunities during the next week to complete three real-life tasks. You are going to test yourself and learn how to dance with the dragons.

## 1. THE CRAVING INTERCEPT

The next time you feel a strong, urgent craving – for sugar, carbs or anything – you are going to treat it like a bomb you need to defuse. You will not give in, but also you will not ignore it. You will go through the full craving decision sequence (see page 211).

**The action:** Hydrate. Pause. Protein anchor if needed.

If it's emotional, use a stress script for just five minutes. Your goal is to meet the panic with a plan and prove to yourself that a craving is just a signal, not a command.

## 2. THE INNER CRITIC FIGHT

The next time you hear that negative whispering saying that you're lazy or you've made mistakes, your mission is to talk back to it. Out loud.

**The action:** Say, 'No. That's the old story,' and then immediately replace it with one of your new coaching phrases.

For example: 'My story is that I'm a person who is getting stronger every day, and my only job is to focus on my next best choice.' You are asserting your authority over the gremlin in your head.

## 3. THE ENERGY BOUNDARY

Your mission is to find one opportunity this week to set a boundary that protects your physical or emotional energy. This is about honouring your body's limits in a social or professional setting.

**The action:** Prove that your wellbeing is not up for negotiation.

This could be saying no to a last-minute request you don't have the capacity for. It could be leaving a party 30 minutes earlier than everyone else because your social battery is dead. It could be using your 'smile and deflect' script to shut down an uncomfortable conversation about your food choices.

## TROUBLESHOOTING

**If your gremlin says:** 'This sounds stressful. I don't want to be looking for problems all week.'
**Your response:** 'I'm not looking for problems; I'm looking for opportunities. This isn't a test I can fail. It's a practice session. A pilot knows you don't learn to handle turbulence by avoiding it; you learn by flying through it in a simulator. This week is my simulator.'

**If your gremlin says:** 'But I haven't had any huge cravings this week. I can't do the challenge.'
**Your response:** 'Perfect. Let's practise on a small one. The next time I feel a small urge for something sweet in the evening, I'll run the full protocol. That way I'll be prepped when a big craving hits me.'

**If your gremlin says:** 'Talking back to myself out loud is crazy.'
**Your response:** 'What's crazy is letting an internal bully run the show for my entire life. This isn't a conversation; it's an eviction notice. I am reclaiming this headspace.'

## YOUR MISSION DEBRIEF

On the morning of day 8, you're going to create a powerful new document. Open a notebook on a fresh page and title it 'My Resilience CV'. Underneath, you are going to log your experience from the last seven days. This is not a diary entry. This is a record of your skills and accomplishments, like a real CV.

## SKILL 1: CRAVING DEFUSAL EXAMPLE

**The situation:** 'Felt a huge urge to eat the office doughnuts at 4 p.m.'

**The action:** 'I left the room, drank a full glass of water and ate the apple and almonds I had in my bag. The craving passed in 10 minutes.'

**The outcome:** 'I felt calm, in control and proud. Proved I am not at the mercy of my cravings.'

## SKILL 2: INNER CRITIC MANAGEMENT EXAMPLE

**The situation:** 'My inner critic told me I was lazy for only doing a 15-minute walk.'

**The action:** 'I said out loud, "No, a powerhouse is someone who shows up, and I showed up today."'

**The outcome:** 'The guilty feeling disappeared. Felt empowered.'

## SKILL 3: BOUNDARY SETTING EXAMPLE

**The situation:** 'Was asked to take on an extra project when I was already drowning.'

**The action:** 'I used a graceful: "I'd love to help, but my plate is too full to give that the attention it deserves right now."'

**The outcome:** 'Felt a bit uncomfortable for 5 seconds and then felt an enormous wave of relief.'

This is now the first page of your resilience CV. You are no longer a rookie. You have documented, real-world experience in handling the hard stuff. This is the proof that you are becoming truly unbreakable.

# CHAPTER 12
# TRAVEL, PARTIES AND REAL LIFE

We've all been there. You're packing for a holiday, feeling pretty good about yourself. You've been consistent, you're feeling strong and you make a promise to your reflection in the mirror: 'This time, it will be different. I'll have the cocktail, but I'll skip the bread basket. I'll enjoy myself, but I won't go completely off the rails.' You are Pre-Holiday You. She is organised. She is optimistic.

She is a delusional liar.

Because the second your foot hits the warm tarmac and you get a whiff of that holiday air, a switch flips. Holiday You arrives. And Holiday You thinks Pre-Holiday You is a bit of a bore.

It starts with an innocent poolside margarita at 11 a.m. (because, you know, you're on holiday). That margarita is followed by a plate of chips. Suddenly, the voice in your head doesn't say, 'Okay, let's have a healthy dinner to balance it out.' It says, 'Well, after that, I might as well order the pizza. And the dessert. We'll start again tomorrow.'

This is the cycle, isn't it? The same thing happens at Christmas, at a week-long work conference or even just a boozy weekend wedding. You go in with the best intentions, but one small deviation from the 'plan' makes you feel like you've failed. And once you feel like a failure, the 'might as well' monster takes over. You think, 'I've already messed up, so I might as well go all in.'

As we saw in chapter 7, the problem isn't your environment. The problem was your plan. It was a simple pass-or-fail test. You were either being 'good' or 'bad'. There was no in-between, so the second you did something 'bad', you just decided you'd failed the whole day and might as well give up completely.

This chapter is about ripping up that ridiculous test paper for good. We are going to create a simple, flexible playbook: a set of strategies so robust and realistic that they can survive a hotel breakfast buffet, a seven-hour flight delay and even a three-day-long party. This is where you learn to bend without breaking. This is where you stop seeing your life as a series of tests you're destined to fail and start seeing it as the place where you actually get to practise your new skills.

## YOUR DAILY SURVIVAL HANDBAG KIT

For your everyday bag, keep a small protein bar (look for 15g+ protein, minimal sugar) and a small pack of nuts. These are your 'never caught hungry' insurance policy for unexpected delays, long meetings, or when lunch gets pushed back.

## YOUR TRAVEL SURVIVAL KIT

Let's be honest, not all travel is created equal. A week sipping cocktails by a pool, a trip back home for a family wedding where your grandma thinks you're 'looking a bit thin', and a three-day work conference in a beige hotel with questionable buffet options are all completely different scenarios. Each one comes with its own unique set of challenges, temptations and emotional landmines.

The old 'pass-or-fail' you would have treated them all the same: a test she was probably going to fail.

The new you with the playbook? She goes in with a strategy. And that strategy starts before you've even zipped up your suitcase.

It starts with packing a small, non-negotiable 'travel survival kit'. This isn't about being a saint; it's about being smart. It's about having options, so you don't end up making a bad decision at 10 p.m. in an airport because the only thing open is a fast-food restaurant.

## PACKING LIST

This is your baseline. Throw these few things in your bag for any trip, no matter where you're going. Better yet, put them all in their own bag that you can put in your suitcase whenever you're going away.

**A few sachets of protein powder:** A quick protein shake made with water or milk in your hotel room is a million times better than starting your day with a sad, sugary pastry that will leave you hungry in an hour. Just ensure you choose a high-quality protein powder option.

- **What to look for:** Check the ingredients. You want a short list without a load of fillers, gums or artificial sweeteners. Look for brands that have minimal artificial additives. If you're not familiar with ingredient lists, a quick Google search of any unfamiliar ingredients can help you make informed choices.
- **For non-vegans:** A whey protein isolate is usually your best bet. It's typically easier on the stomach than a standard whey concentrate.
- **For vegans:** Look for a blend, usually pea and brown rice protein. This combo gives you a complete amino acid profile. A plain pea protein can sometimes taste a bit earthy.

**Electrolyte/hydration sachets:** Earlier on I warned you that a lot of these are rubbish. And they are. But a good-quality electrolyte sachet has a definite time and place, and that place is a stuffy, dehydrating aeroplane cabin or a sweaty holiday destination. They are a tool. Look for brands that are only sweetened with stevia and have no artificial colours or junk. They are brilliant for energy and stopping those fake 'I'm hungry but I'm actually just thirsty' signals.

**Your favourite teabags:** A small comfort, but a big deal. A peppermint tea can save you from travel-induced bloating, and a chamomile tea can help you unwind in a strange hotel room.

**A reusable water bottle:** Simple, but crucial. You're a hundred times more likely to stay hydrated if you have water with you, and it stops you from buying overpriced, sugar-free drinks out of desperation.

**A couple of your favourite protein bars:** For emergencies only. We're talking flight delays, getting stuck in traffic or arriving at your hotel after the kitchen has closed. Choose one you like the taste of, not one that tastes like flavoured chalk.

### YOUR MENTAL SURVIVAL KIT

The most important survival tool isn't in your suitcase; it's in your head. These are the mindset shifts that will help to keep you sane whilst you're away.

**1. The 'one good choice' rule**

This is your antidote to the 'might as well' monster. The old you would eat a croissant for breakfast and think, 'Well, the day is ruined. I might as well eat pizza for lunch and a whole tiramisu for dinner.'

> The new you follows the 'one good choice' rule. It's simple: focus on making one good choice at your next meal. That's it. Had the croissant for breakfast? Fine. For lunch, focus on finding some protein and veg. You haven't failed. You've just reset.
>
> This rule single-handedly destroys the all-or-nothing cycle.
>
> **2. The scout-ahead tactic**
>
> Anxiety thrives on the unknown. The easiest way to kill travel anxiety is to do a tiny bit of homework beforehand. This isn't about being obsessive; it's about being smart.
>
> Before you go to a restaurant, spend 60 seconds having a quick look at the menu online to plan what your options are.

Now, let's get specific. Here's the game plan for three main types of trip.

# 1. THE HOLIDAY (AKA 'OPERATION ENJOY YOURSELF WITHOUT A MELTDOWN')

**The challenge:** It's the trip you've been looking forward to, and your brain immediately goes into full 'what happens on holiday, stays on holiday' mode. The danger isn't the one cocktail; it's the one cocktail convincing you that the entire week is now a nutritional write-off.

**Your game plan:**
- **The mindset:** The goal is balance, not to be a saint. You are, of course, going to have the local speciality and the glass of wine. This is not about deprivation. The strategy is to anchor your days with good choices.
- **The tactic:** Start your day with a protein-focused breakfast (this is where your protein powder sachet might come in handy if

the buffet is just carbs). This sets your blood sugar for the day and stops you from being ravenously hungry by 11 a.m. Then, go and enjoy your lunch, your dinner, your cocktail. You've created a stable foundation, so the rest can be flexible.

## 2. THE FAMILY GATHERING
## (WHEN YOUR NEW HABITS MEET OLD EXPECTATIONS)

**The challenge:** You've been eating well for weeks, feeling confident in your new routine. Then you arrive at your mum's house and she's made your 'favourite' lasagna, insisting you have seconds because 'you look thin'. Your sister comments that you're 'being difficult' when you bring your own snacks, and suddenly you're 12 years old again, seeking approval through your plate.

**Your game plan:**
- **The mindset:** You're not rejecting their love – you're protecting your progress. Food is not the only way to show care or receive it.
- **The tactic:** Use the 'compliment and redirect' technique: 'Mum, this smells incredible and I can see how much effort you put in. I'm going to have a smaller portion because I had a big lunch, but tell me about this recipe – is it Grandma's?' This acknowledges their effort while maintaining your boundaries. Have your response ready for pushback: 'I'm learning to listen to my body better these days. It's actually quite liberating!' Say it with genuine enthusiasm – make it about your growth, not their inadequacy.

## 3. THE WORK TRIP (AKA 'THE BEIGE BUFFET BATTLE')

**The challenge:** Boredom, exhaustion and terrible corporate catering. It's the sad pastries at the morning meeting, the greasy, beige lunch buffet and the lonely evening in a hotel room where the minibar Pringles start calling your name.

**Your game plan:**
- **The mindset:** Your goal is to fuel your brain and body so you can perform well, not to use food as entertainment or a cure for loneliness.
- **The tactic:** Create your own 'hotel room stash'. Have your protein powder for breakfast. Keep your emergency protein bars on hand. If you can, pop to a local supermarket when you arrive and grab some Greek yogurts for the mini-fridge, some nuts, some fruit. Having your own options means you can navigate the beige buffet strategically, focusing on the protein and salad, without feeling deprived or ending up eating three spring rolls out of sheer desperation.

## NAVIGATING THE TRICKY ZONES: BREAKFAST BUFFETS, AIRPORTS AND ROOM SERVICE

These are the places where plans go to die. But it doesn't have to be this way. With a few simple strategies, you can navigate these zones like a pro. This isn't about having superhuman willpower; it's about having a better game plan.

### SURVIVING THE AIRPORT DAY

Airports are food deserts designed by people who hate you. The options are almost always overpriced, unhealthy and underwhelming. This is where your scout-ahead tactic and your survival kit become your best friends, so you can avoid making panicked decisions.

1. **Eat a real meal before you go:** Never, ever arrive at the airport hungry. Have a proper, protein-packed meal at home before you leave. This puts you in control. If you're taking an early flight, see the next step.
2. **Pack your own snacks:** Your emergency protein bar is for this exact moment. Having one in your bag is the difference between feeling calm and feeling desperate. An apple and a small bag of nuts are also brilliant options.
3. **Hydrate, hydrate, hydrate:** Fill up your reusable water bottle the second you get through security. Dehydration feels like hunger. A lot of the time when you're craving junk in an airport, your body is just screaming for water.
4. **If you *have* to buy food:** Look for the pre-made salads with chicken or egg, protein pots or Greek yogurt. Yes, it's boring, but it will make you feel a million times better than a greasy slice of pizza.

## YOUR IN-FLIGHT SURVIVAL KIT (FOR LONG-HAUL FLIGHTS)

Airline food ranges from bland to inedible, especially on long flights. Pack these flight-friendly options that won't get confiscated at security:

- **Protein bars or protein powder sachets** (mix with water you buy after security).
- **Hard-boiled eggs** (make them at home the night before).
- **Cheese sticks or wrapped, small-portion cheeses.**
- **Dried chickpeas or edamame** (nut-free protein option).
- **Apple slices with individual almond butter packets** (if nuts are allowed on your flight).
- **Protein-rich crackers**, like chickpea or lentil-based options.
- **Homemade energy balls** made with seeds instead of nuts.

## JET LAG: YOUR SLEEP SALVAGE PLAYBOOK

Jet lag scrambles your internal clock, leaving you exhausted but wired, craving quick energy fixes that'll only make things worse. Here's how to get your body back on track without derailing your progress.

### *The pre-flight prep*

- **Hydrate aggressively:** I know I sound like a broken record, but this is crucial. The dry air on a plane is brutally dehydrating, which makes every symptom of jet lag ten times worse. Drink water regularly.

### *The in-flight strategy*

- **Sleep according to the new time zone:** Adjust your watch to your new time zone ASAP. If it's nighttime where you're going, you need to try to sleep. Use your eye mask, your earplugs, your neck pillow. Do whatever it takes. If it's daytime where you're going, try to stay awake. Watch films, read a book. You are trying to trick your body into the new rhythm.

### *Your in-flight frenemies: caffeine and alcohol*

- **The alcohol rule:** If you are going to have a drink, have one. Then, for every alcoholic drink you have, you must have two full glasses of water. Alcohol is brutally dehydrating and will make your jet lag a thousand times worse, so you need to actively counteract it.
- **The coffee rule:** Coffee is not a crutch; it is a strategic tool. Use it with intention: no caffeine after 2 p.m. in your destination's time zone. If you land in the morning and need to stay awake, one or two coffees before 2 p.m. can be a lifesaver. Anything after that, and you are sabotaging your chances of sleeping that night.

### Your on-arrival sleep salvage kit

- **Get into the light:** If you arrive during the day, get outside into the sunlight for at least 20 minutes. The natural light hits your eyes and sends a powerful signal to your brain's internal clock to reset. It is the most powerful jet-lag cure on the planet.
- **Move your body:** Go for a 15- to 20-minute brisk walk. It will get your blood flowing, boost your energy and help your body understand that it's 'active time'.
- **Anchor your meals to the new time zone:** Eat your meals at the correct local time. Even if you're not hungry for dinner at 4 p.m., have a small, protein-rich meal. This helps to anchor your body's internal clock.
- **The strategic nap = a dangerous game:** If you absolutely must nap, there are two rules.
  **Rule 1:** Keep it short; 20–30 minutes, max. Set an alarm. A short power nap can be restorative. A long, two-hour nap will destroy your chances of sleeping that night.
  **Rule 2:** No napping after 3 p.m. local time. Ever.

### The first night's sleep: your secret weapons

This is the big one. Getting a decent sleep on the first night is the key to winning the war against jet lag.

- **Eat a carb-heavy dinner:** This is the time to use your 'strategic carb' lever. A meal with some smart carbs (sweet potatoes, quinoa or oats) can help raise serotonin and make you feel sleepy.
- **Your sleep supporters:** A magnesium glycinate supplement before bed can help relax your muscles and your mind. Chamomile tea is also your best friend.
- **Make your room a cave:** Total darkness. Cool temperature. No screens for an hour before you want to sleep. You have to give your brain every possible signal that it is time to shut down.

## HOW TO WIN AT THE HOTEL BREAKFAST BUFFET

The hotel breakfast buffet is a sugar trap. It's a sea of processed carbs designed to make you forget what a proper meal looks like. Your old 'all-or-nothing' self would either try to be perfect and have a single, sad piece of fruit, or say 'Sod it' and pile her plate with three different kinds of beige foods.

The new you is a strategist. You do one simple thing first: walk a lap before you pick up a plate.

Seriously. Don't just grab a plate and start loading it at the first station. Do a full 360-degree scan of the entire buffet. You're on a mission. You are looking for one thing and one thing only: the protein station.

1. **Start with protein:** Get a generous serving of eggs. If there are other protein options like Greek yogurt (the real, thick stuff, not the sugary fruit-corner nonsense), smoked salmon or some ham, grab those, too. This is the foundation of your plate.
2. **Add colour:** Now look for any fruit or veggies. Sliced tomatoes, mushrooms, spinach at the omelette station, or a bowl of berries.
3. **The insurance policy:** If the buffet is a total disaster and the scrambled eggs look suspiciously like yellow soup, this is when you deploy your travel survival kit. Go back to your room, mix your protein sachet with water or coffee, and have that with a piece of fruit from the buffet.

Job done. You've won.

## THE ROOM SERVICE EDIT

You've had a long day. You're exhausted. You're alone in your room and the thought of putting on real clothes and stepping out to find food is just too much. Room service is calling your name. The temptation is to order the big, comforting club sandwich with a mountain of chips or the stodgy pasta, but you can find healthy options on the menu and make simple edits.

1. **Ignore the obvious:** Scan past the sandwiches and pasta sections. They are rarely your friend. Look for the main courses or grill section.
2. **Look for the magic words:** 'Grilled', 'Steamed', 'Roasted', or 'Seared'. You're searching for a simple piece of protein. A grilled chicken breast, a piece of salmon, a steak.
3. **Make the edit:** This is the crucial part. The dish will probably come with chips or potatoes. When you order, make one simple request: 'Could I please swap the chips for extra steamed vegetables or a side salad?'
4. **The result:** You will get a delicious, satisfying, protein-and-veg-packed meal delivered right to your door. It will feel like a total treat, but it will be a meal that serves your body and your goals. This simple swap is a total power move.

## THE RESTAURANT PLAYBOOK: YOUR SIMPLE GUIDE TO ORDERING ANYTHING

Ah, the restaurant menu. That beautiful document that can send a sane person into a spiral of anxiety. You know the feeling. The menu arrives. It's the size of a novel. Your friends are all excitedly choosing the pasta or the chips, and your heart starts to beat a little faster. The internal monologue begins: 'Okay, I should get the salad. But that's so boring. The steak looks good, but it comes with that creamy sauce and a mountain of fries. Maybe the fish? Oh god, it's battered. Okay, salad it is. Again.'

Or, the alternative monologue: 'Sod it. I'm out for dinner. I'm getting the burger AND the chips AND we're splitting that chocolate fudge cake. I'll just start again tomorrow.'

Sound familiar? It's the old pass-or-fail test, live and in person. Well, we're ripping up that test paper. From now on, you're going into every restaurant with a new, dead simple playbook. It's not a diet rule. It's a strategy for freedom.

## THE 'PICK TWO' PRINCIPLE

Let's start to build our restaurant playbook. It's incredibly simple. When you look at the main course menu, you have three categories to choose from. Your job is to pick two to prioritise.

1. **PROTEIN:** A solid serving of the good stuff (the chicken, steak, fish, lentils, tofu, etc.). This is your anchor. It keeps you full and your blood sugar stable.
2. **VEG:** A decent amount of colour. (The salad, the roasted broccoli, the green beans.) This is for fibre, nutrients and filling you up.
3. **FUN:** This is the other stuff. The stuff that makes a meal feel like a real treat. (The wine or cocktail, chips, the creamy pasta, the rich sauce, the bread, the extra cheese.)

You don't get to have a massive portion of all three. That's not a meal; that's a food coma. You just get to pick two. Let me show you how it works in the wild.

## THE 'PICK TWO' PRINCIPLE IN ACTION

### Scenario 1: You choose PROTEIN + VEG

This is your classic, smart, feel-good choice. You're at a steakhouse. You order the steak (PROTEIN) and you use your room-service edit trick: 'Could I please have that with the side salad instead of the chips?' The salad is your VEG.

**The result:** You have a delicious, satisfying meal. You leave feeling full and energised, not bloated and sleepy. You still feel like you've had a proper restaurant meal, but you've nailed your two priorities: protein and vegetables.

### Scenario 2: You choose PROTEIN + FUN

It's been a long week, and you really, really want the chips. Or the pasta. Fine. Let's do it. You're at that Italian place. You see a beautiful chicken pasta dish. The chicken is your PROTEIN. The pasta is your FUN.

**The result:** You order the pasta. You enjoy every single bite of it. And you consciously decide not to order the giant side salad *and* the cheesy garlic bread to go with it. You've made a strategic choice. You prioritised the thing you really wanted (the pasta) and the thing your body needs (the chicken). It's a trade-off, not a tragedy.

### Scenario 3: You choose VEG + FUN

This is a less common choice for a main meal, but it's a great strategy. Maybe you're at a pizza place. You know the pizza is going to be your FUN. So, you decide your other priority is VEG.

**The result:** You order a veggie-loaded pizza instead of the double pepperoni with extra cheese. And you have a big side salad with it. You've still had the pizza you were craving, but you've cleverly dialled up the veg and fibre, which will make you feel a hundred times better afterwards.

See how this works? It's a conscious choice. You are in the driver's seat. It's not about restriction; it's about strategy.

'But!' I hear you cry. 'A meal is more than just the main course!' and you're right. While the 'Pick Two' principle is your secret weapon for the main course, here's how you apply the same playbook to the rest of the dining experience, so you feel in control from the moment you sit down to the moment you leave.

## THE SMARTER STARTER STRATEGY

The danger with starters is filling up on deep-fried, beige rubbish before your main course even arrives. The goal is to have a little something to take the edge off your hunger, not to eat a whole second meal.

- **Your game plan:** Look for a starter that is either protein- or veg-based.
- **What it looks like:** Prawns, scallops, a caprese salad, chicken skewers, a simple soup. These are all smart choices. What you're trying to avoid is the giant, shareable platter of deep-fried everything or the massive basket of cheesy garlic bread.

## THE DRINK DEAL

Let's be real, a glass of wine or a cocktail is often part of the fun of eating out. That's totally fine. We just need to account for it in our playbook.

- **Your game plan:** Acknowledge that your drinks are part of your FUN choice for the evening. This helps you make a conscious trade-off.

- **What it looks like:** If you know you're going to have a couple of glasses of wine (FUN), don't compound it by pairing it with more fun food like pizza or pasta. Instead, use that as your guide when choosing your main course – prioritise PROTEIN + VEG like steak and salad. You get your wine enjoyment without the food hangover.

## THE DESSERT DILEMMA

This is the big one. This is often where the 'all or nothing' monster comes out to play. You've had a great meal, and then the dessert menu arrives and your brain goes wild.

- **Your game plan:** Introduce the 'two-bite tactic'. This is a game-changer.
- **How it works:** Order one dessert that you share. Take two proper, mindful, glorious bites of that sticky toffee pudding or chocolate lava cake. Savour them completely. You get the full taste, the full experience, and the full satisfaction without the waste or expense. What you'll find is that those first two bites give you 90 per cent of the pleasure anyway – the rest would just be mindless eating. Plus, sharing creates a lovely social moment rather than individual food guilt.

    If you're dining alone, simply ask your server about their most popular dessert and request 'a small taste portion' if possible. Many restaurants are happy to accommodate this, especially when you explain you just want to experience their signature dish. Or scout the menu beforehand and choose a restaurant that offers smaller dessert portions or dessert-tasting options.

- **The 'share and conquer' tactic:** Even better. Order one dessert for the table with a few spoons. You can all have your two glorious bites, and then it's gone. It's a shared experience, not a solo sugar binge. You get the fun without the food coma.

## EXTRA PRO-TIPS FOR YOUR PLAYBOOK

- **The bread basket standoff:** If the bread basket is your personal kryptonite, just ask the waiter to take it away. It's not rude. It's you being smart. Out of sight equals out of mind.
- **The vegetable swap:** If your meal is looking a bit beige because you went for the PROTEIN + FUN option (like steak and chips), ask if you can swap the chips for vegetables or salad instead. Most restaurants are happy to do this at no extra cost, and you're still sticking to your two categories while getting more nutrition.
- **The menu scout:** Look at the menu online before you go. This removes the pressure of making a quick decision while hungry and surrounded by tempting options. You can make your 'Pick Two' choice calmly at home.
- **Sauce on the side:** A simple piece of grilled salmon is a great choice. The same piece of salmon drowning in a creamy, buttery sauce is a different story. Asking for the sauce on the side puts you in control. You can just add a little bit for flavour, rather than have your entire meal swimming in it.

This playbook puts you back in charge. You can now walk into any restaurant, with any menu, and feel calm and confident that you can make a choice that serves both your body and your happiness.

## WEDDINGS, BUFFETS AND BIG WEEKENDS: SOCIAL SURVIVAL TIPS

Let's talk about the special parties. A wedding, for example. You've bought the new outfit, you've got the fancy shoes on and you feel great. You walk into the reception, grab a glass of prosecco and then it begins. The slow, silent ambush of the canapés. Tiny, deep-fried things start appearing from every direction. Before you know it, you've eaten four mini sausage rolls and something involving goat's cheese and the internal monologue starts screaming: 'I've blown it before the starter has even been served! Sod it. Let's just go for it.'

Weddings, big birthday weekends and family get-togethers are not a single meal. They are a marathon of social eating. They can easily dismantle your best intentions. So, let's give you a playbook to deal with them. Once again, this isn't about restriction. It's about being the savvy, strategic guest who has an amazing time and leaves without a food coma and a week-long guilt hangover.

## THE PRE-GAME PREP: YOUR MENTAL WARM-UP

The battle is won or lost before you even start. How you mentally prepare for the event is everything.

- **Ditch the 'last meal' mentality:** This is the single biggest mistake people make. They 'save themselves' for a big event by starving all day. This is a catastrophic plan. You will arrive ravenous, your blood sugar will be in the gutter and you will have zero control. You will eat everything that isn't nailed down.
  **The power move:** Eat a normal, protein-packed breakfast or lunch. Have a big chicken salad or some eggs before you go. Arriving at an event feeling stable and satisfied, not starving, is your secret weapon. It puts you in charge.
- **Decide what's 'worth it':** Not all food at a party is created equal. There are the dry, boring mini quiches, and then there is the incredible, triple-chocolate wedding cake that your best friend spent months choosing. They do not hold the same value.

**The power move:** Set your intention before you go, not your specific choice. Tell yourself: 'I'm going to enjoy this party, and I'm going to have one treat that really speaks to me when I see what's on offer.' This could be Grandma's famous tiramisu, the birthday cake, or those fancy canapés – whatever looks most special when you arrive. The key is making one conscious, regret-free choice rather than having a bit of everything.

## THE EVENT PLAYBOOK

You arrive. Tempting food choices are everywhere. Here's how you navigate it.

- **The canapé strategy:** Those bite-sized temptations floating past can derail you fast.
  
  **The power move:** Set yourself a canapé limit before you start drinking or socialising – say, three canapés, maximum. Choose them consciously rather than mindlessly grabbing whatever passes by. Look for the ones with actual protein (smoked salmon, chicken, cheese) rather than just pastry and carbs.
- **The two-bite tactic for special treats:** As we've seen, this is your secret weapon for the 'worth it' moment. Whether it's the wedding cake, the dessert buffet, or your grandma's legendary tiramisu.
  
  **The result:** You've had the cake. You've participated. You've enjoyed it. And all without needing to eat a slab the size of your head. It is the ultimate act of having your cake and eating it, too.
- **The late-night food question:** The bacon butties or pizza slices appear at 10 p.m. It's tempting. Before you grab one, ask yourself one simple question: 'Am I actually hungry?' Generally, you're just tired, a bit drunk or eating it because it's there.

If you're genuinely hungry, fine. But if not, have a glass of water and feel smug about the decision you'll be very happy with in the morning.

This playbook isn't about being the 'good' one at the party. It's about being the *smart* one. The one who can fully enjoy the celebration without the physical or emotional hangover.

## THE NEXT-DAY RESET: HOW TO RE-BALANCE YOURSELF

The party was fun. But you wake up the next day feeling a bit fuzzy, a bit bloated, and with the faint taste of wedding cake mixed with regret in your mouth. This is a critical moment. The old you had two options:

1. **The punisher:** 'Right, that's it. I'm having nothing but green juice and misery today to make up for it.'
2. **The enabler:** 'The weekend's a write-off. Might as well order a massive greasy breakfast and keep going.'

Both are terrible choices. Your mission today is not to punish yourself, nor is it to continue the binge. Your mission is simply to get back to normal. Here is your simple, three-step reset plan:

- **Hydrate like a pro:** Before you do anything else, drink a huge glass of water, maybe with one of your electrolyte sachets in it. You are dehydrated from the booze, the dancing and the salty food. Hydration is your number one priority.
- **Anchor your next meal with protein:** Do not skip breakfast. Do not have a 'light' breakfast of just toast. Go right back to your playbook. Have a proper meal, anchored with protein. Scrambled eggs are perfect. This will stabilise your blood sugar and shut down the cravings that are screaming for more beige food.

- **Move your body gently:** The last thing you probably feel like doing is a brutal workout. And you shouldn't opt for it either. The goal isn't to punish yourself by 'burning off' the cake. The goal is to help your body feel normal again. The best thing you can do is go for a 20- to 30-minute walk, preferably outside. It will do wonders for your digestion, your mood and your energy levels.

That's it. Water, protein, walk. By lunchtime, you will feel a million times better. You've proven to yourself that one fun night doesn't have to derail your entire week. You just reset and carry on. This is what true food freedom feels like.

## THE CONDENSED PLAYBOOK

We've navigated a minefield of real-life situations in this chapter. If it felt like a lot, don't worry. Here's everything you need to remember on one simple page. This is your new travel and social playbook.

- **Pack your travel survival kit.** A few key items (good-quality protein powder, electrolytes, your favourite tea) make up your insurance policy against bad food environments.
- **Use the 'one good choice' rule.** Had a pastry for breakfast? Fine. Just focus on making one good choice at lunch. This rule single-handedly kills the 'all-or-nothing' cycle.
- **Master the buffet.** First, walk a lap. Next find the protein. Then follow the simple equation: Half your plate = protein; the other half = colour. Then add a spoonful of fun if you want to.
- **Use the 'pick two' restaurant tactic.** Prioritise two out of three categories for your main course: protein, veg or fun. This gives you strategic freedom without the guilt.

- **Deploy the 'two-bite rule' for dessert.** Share a dessert and savour two mindful, glorious bites of the cake or dessert you really want. It gives you all the pleasure without the food coma.
- **Survive social pressure with a script.** If someone comments on your food choices, just smile, agree and deflect.
- **Reset the day after.** The morning after a big event is not for punishment or panic. Your simple reset: water, protein and a gentle walk.

# YOUR TWELFTH ACTION PLAN: MAKING SMART CHOICES

**The mindset shift:** The goal isn't to punish yourself by 'burning off' a binge. The goal is to help your body feel normal again.

**The goal:** Build confidence and maintain your progress when life takes you outside your normal routine – whether that's holidays, work trips, social events, or just being unexpectedly busy.

**The task:** Create 'habit anchors' that travel with you. Your usual environment supports your new habits. You know where the good snacks are, your meal timing works and your routine feels natural. But the moment you're somewhere different – a hotel, a friend's house, a work conference – suddenly you feel like you're starting from scratch.

**What goes in your wallet**

- A small card with 3 non-negotiable habits (e.g., 'Protein at every meal', 'Water first', 'Walk after eating').
- Emergency snack (so you're not hunting for vending machines when hungry).
- Screenshot of your 'flexible wins' list (small victories that count no matter where you are).
- Photo of your favourite healthy meal (visual reminder when scanning unfamiliar menus).

**The practice**

- When you're feeling uncertain in a new environment, pull out these anchors and ask: 'Which of my three habits can I easily maintain here?'

- Even if you can only manage one (like having protein at breakfast), you're still moving forward. Progress over perfection, always.
- The point isn't to be perfect in unfamiliar situations – it's to prove to yourself that your healthy habits aren't dependent on perfect conditions.

You now have a helpful playbook to set you up for almost any scenario. You have practical strategies to make you feel confident at a wedding, on holiday or travelling. But let's be brutally honest. Sometimes, you're not going to follow the playbook. Sometimes, life gets too much. You're too tired, too sad or too fed up to be strategic. Sometimes having a small portion of dessert will turn into the whole cake. And that's okay. Because you are human.

The old you would let that one meal turn into a week-long spiral of guilt and bad choices. But the new you? The new you has a plan that stops the spiral in its tracks. So, what happens when the plan goes completely out of the window and you eat the whole pizza?

Let's talk about the 24-hour reset.

## CHAPTER 13

# BACK ON TRACK IN 24 HOURS

So ... you ate the whole pizza. Or maybe it wasn't a pizza; maybe it was half a birthday cake, a family-sized bag of Doritos, or a full-scale assault on the hotel minibar. Whatever it was, it happened. The plan went out the window. And now it's the morning after and you're spiralling.

Let's just sit with that feeling for a second, because we all know it intimately. It's not just the physical stuff – the bloating, the slight headache, the feeling that you're 90 per cent dry bread and melted cheese – it's the mental gymnastics that are the real killer. The voice in your head is having a field day. It's loud, it's smug and it's saying things like:

- 'See? I knew you couldn't do it.'
- 'You've completely ruined all your hard work.'
- 'You have zero self-control. What's wrong with you?'

First, take a deep breath. You are not broken. You have not failed. You have not 'ruined everything'. You're human, and humans sometimes eat pizza.

Here's what I want you to remember: the person who binged last night and the person who's reading this right now are the same person. You didn't transform into a different, weaker version of yourself because you ate some food. You're still the same intelligent, capable you who's been making progress. One meal – even a really big, messy meal – doesn't erase all the good choices you've made, or the knowledge you've gained.

The truth is this: every single person who has ever successfully changed their relationship with food has had nights like this. The difference between the people who succeed and the people who give up isn't that the successful ones never mess up – it's that they get back on track quickly, without drama, and without punishing themselves.

You're about to prove to yourself that you're one of the people who gets back up. You're about to show yourself that one difficult night doesn't define you. You've got this. You've always had this. Now let's get you feeling like yourself again.

I'm going to give you a simple, calm, step-by-step protocol to get you back to feeling like yourself in 24 hours. This is not a punishment. It is not a detox or a cleanse. There are no weird juices or miserable fasts involved.

Think of this chapter as your reset button. It's a series of gentle, powerful actions designed to stabilise your blood sugar, calm your inflammation and, most importantly, quiet the nasty voice in your head. This is how you prove to yourself that one off-plan meal is just that: one meal. It's a data point, not a disaster. It doesn't define you, and it certainly doesn't derail you. Not anymore.

## THE STOP-THE-SLIDE PROTOCOL

So, that pizza scenario ... Let's pick up where we left off.

You're waking up feeling physically bloated from the pizza and mentally beaten up as you start sliding down the spiral. The little gremlin in your head is screaming, telling you that you've ruined everything and the only solution is to either starve yourself or just give up and eat a croissant.

As you'll know by now, our first job is to politely tell that gremlin to shut up.

Our second job is to follow an incredibly simple, three-step protocol.

## YOUR FIRST 90 MINUTES: A STEP-BY-STEP GUIDE

This is not a punishment. Your mission for the next few hours is not to 'fix the damage' – it's simply to get back on track and stop the slide. That's it. You just need do these three things.

### Step 1: Salt water elixir

Before you do anything else, you are going to drink one big glass of water.

**What it is:** A pint of water with a pinch of unrefined sea salt. Not freezing cold, just cool. Or if you have an electrolyte sachet, use that instead of the sea salt.

**Why it works:** You think you feel rubbish because of the pizza. But you feel rubbish because you are desperately dehydrated. The pizza was probably loaded with salt, and if you had any booze, that's made it even worse. Dehydration is making you feel foggy, sluggish and headachy, and it's making the bloating a thousand times worse. This one glass of water starts to rehydrate your system, helps your body start flushing out the excess salt, and wakes up your digestion. It is the kindest and most powerful first move you can make.

## Step 2: Go on one walk

I know, I know. The last thing you feel like doing is putting on a pair of leggings and moving your tired, bloated body. Your brain is telling you to stay inside on the sofa. But we are not going for a punishing workout. This is a non-negotiable, gentle walk.

**What it is:** A 15 to 20-minute walk. Outside, if you can possibly manage it. This is not a power walk. It is not a run. It is a slow, head-clearing stroll. You don't have to feel like it; you just have to do it.

**Why it works:** This walk is your secret weapon for two reasons. Physically, it does something magical for your blood sugar. After a big carb-heavy meal, a gentle walk helps your muscles soak up the excess sugar from your bloodstream without needing a huge insulin spike, which stops the energy crash and cravings later. Mentally, it gets you out of the house and stops you from sitting inside, wallowing in guilt. The fresh air and daylight will do more for your mood than anything else. It's a physical signal to your brain that you are moving on.

## Step 3: Prepare one Gold Plate

This is your reset meal. Not a sad 'punishment' meal. Not a continuation of the binge. We're going to call it your Gold Plate because it is the most valuable meal of your week.

**What it is:** A plate that is loaded with three things: protein, fibre and healthy fats. That's it. Notice what's not on there: a load of heavy, starchy carbs or sugar. We're giving your digestion a break and focusing on nutrients.

**What it looks like in real life:**
- **Breakfast option:** Two or three scrambled eggs (protein/fat) cooked in a bit of butter, with a side of spinach or half an avocado (veg/fat).

- **Lunch/dinner option:** A big salad (colour) with a grilled chicken breast or fish or tofu (protein) and a simple olive oil dressing (fat).

**Why it works:** This meal is a direct message to your body and your brain. The protein and healthy fats will stabilise your blood sugar, which shuts down the gremlin screaming for more carbs and sugar. The fibre from the vegetables helps your digestion get back to normal. Mentally, eating a plate full of nourishing, satisfying food proves to you, in real time, that you are back in control. You haven't failed. You've just had your reset meal, and now you're back on track.

That's the protocol. One glass, one walk, one Gold Plate. By the time you've done these three simple things, you will feel physically lighter, mentally clearer and the slide will have been completely stopped in its tracks.

## YOUR NO-NONSENSE FAQs

### *'Okay, but can I have my coffee?'*
Yes! But here's the deal: water first, then coffee. The one glass of water is non-negotiable and must come first to rehydrate you. After that, absolutely have your coffee. Just try to have it with your Gold Plate meal, not on an empty stomach, to be kinder to your blood sugar.

### *'What if I'm not hungry for the Gold Plate meal?'*
Then don't force it. The protocol is about listening to your body, not punishing it. Honour your lack of hunger but make a promise to yourself: a Gold Plate will be the next thing you eat when you *do* get hungry. Don't let your first meal of the day be a handful of

crackers at 3 p.m. Wait for your hunger signals and then have your proper reset meal.

### 'Should I track my calories today to see the damage?'

Your only job today is to follow the protocol: water, walk, Gold Plate. That's it. Tomorrow you simply return to your regular mindful-eating approach – no punishment, no restriction, just back to taking good care of yourself.

### 'Should I weigh myself to assess the fallout?'

You'll notice this book doesn't focus on the bathroom scales. That's intentional. Your weight fluctuates daily based on water retention, hormones, digestion and countless other factors that have nothing to do with your actual progress. We're measuring success by how you feel, how strong you're getting, and how confident you become in your relationship with food.

## YOUR 24-HOUR RESET CHECKLIST

You've done the hard part. You've completed the stop-the-slide protocol and you've broken the cycle of panic. Now we need a simple timeline for the rest of the day. No big decisions, no complicated rules. You just follow the checklist. The goal is simple: by the time your head hits the pillow tonight, you will feel physically better, calm and mentally back in charge.

### 1. THE A.M. PLAN: THE MORNING RESET

**The stop-the-slide protocol.** One glass, one walk, one Gold Plate. The most important part of your day is already behind you. Give yourself a little nod of acknowledgement for that. Say to yourself:

'My old self would be punishing myself right now. Instead, I chose to be strategic. The hardest part is over.' This reframes the morning as a victory, not a recovery.

**Keep the water coming.** Water is your best friend for the rest of the day. It's helping to flush out the bloating and rehydrate your system. Keep your reusable bottle with you and sip constantly. Don't force it, just make it a priority.

**Coffee: with a rule.** You've had your water. You've had your Gold Plate breakfast. Now you can have your coffee. Having it with or after your food is much kinder to your blood sugar and will help you avoid any extra jitters.

## 2. THE MIDDAY PLAN: LUNCHTIME ANCHOR

**Lunch: second Gold Plate.** This is your anchor meal for the middle of the day. Do not skip this meal. Starving yourself now will only lead to a massive energy crash and a craving-fuelled disaster zone this afternoon. As you eat your lunch, focus on the food. Your thought is: 'This is not a "diet" meal. This is a stability meal. I am giving my body exactly what it needs to feel strong.'

Your lunch should look a lot like your breakfast:

- **Focus:** Protein, colour (veggies) and healthy fats.
- **What it looks like:** A big salad with a salmon fillet and an olive oil dressing. A chicken breast with a huge pile of roasted broccoli. Keep it simple. Keep it nourishing.

## 3. THE P.M. PLAN: NAVIGATING THE AFTERNOON AND EVENING

**The 3 p.m. panic snack.** Around mid-afternoon, you might feel an energy slump. This is the danger zone where the old you would have reached for a biscuit. The new you is prepared. If you feel that dip, have a strategic snack that combines protein and/or fat.

- **What it looks like:** A small handful of almonds, an apple with a spoonful of peanut butter, or a small pot of full-fat Greek yogurt. This will stabilise your blood sugar, not spike it. Before you have your snack, notice the feeling without judgment. 'Okay, I feel an energy dip. This is normal. This is biological, not a moral failing. I have a plan for this.

**Dinner: the final reset.** Your last meal of the day is your final act of self-care. It's another Gold Plate, but we can be clever here to set you up for a great night's sleep.

- **The formula:** Protein + a ton of veggies + a *small* strategic serving of smart carbs.
- **What it looks like:** A piece of grilled fish with a huge portion of green beans, with a few new potatoes on the side. The small serving of carbs can help your brain produce serotonin, making you feel calm and ready for sleep.

**The digital sunset.** Your final mission is to get a good night's sleep. This is non-negotiable. An hour before you plan to go to sleep, your phone and your laptop are done for the day. Your brain has been through enough. The blue light will only mess with your sleep hormones.

**Instead:** Read a book. Have a chamomile tea. Listen to some relaxing music. Tell your brain the day is over. You've successfully completed the reset. Job done.

You're not learning anything new today – you're simply applying the wisdom you've already gained when you need it most.

That's what real progress looks like.

## LANGUAGE SWAP: HOW TO BE KIND WITHOUT LETTING YOURSELF OFF THE HOOK

### BEING KIND TO YOURSELF ISN'T GIVING UP

There's a crucial difference between self-compassion and self-indulgence. Self-compassion says: 'I made a choice I regret, but I'm still a good person and worthy of care. Let me do something loving for my body today.' Self-indulgence says: 'I messed up, so nothing matters anymore, including myself. Pass the biscuits.'

Being kind to yourself means treating yourself like you would treat a good friend who made a mistake. You wouldn't berate them or tell them they're hopeless. You'd help them get back on track with love and practical support. That's exactly what today's protocol does – it's practical kindness in action.

Let's talk about that voice in your head. The morning after you've eaten the whole pizza, that voice is not your friend. It's a cruel, relentless bully. It uses a specific vocabulary.

'You're so weak. You have no willpower.'

'You're disgusting. You failed, again.'

'You're out of control. You've ruined everything.'

This language is not motivational. It is paralysing. It makes you feel both ashamed and hopeless and the easiest thing to do is just give up and eat more rubbish to numb the feeling. The shame fuels the spiral. So, the most powerful part of our 24-hour reset isn't the nourishing food or the walk; it's a conscious language swap.

We are going to fire that internal bully and hire a new inner coach.

Instead of a permissive pushover who says, 'Oh, it doesn't matter, darling, eat whatever you want!', which is just another form of giving up, this fresh approach is kind but firm. Like a good physio, she acknowledges the pain, but she doesn't let you wallow in it. She tells you exactly what you need to do to get strong again. Her job is to be compassionate *without* making excuses.

## YOUR NEW VOCABULARY: FROM CRITIC TO COACH

Here's how we swap the language. Identify the old, bullying thought and consciously replace it with a new, coaching thought.

**Old critic:** 'I failed. I have zero willpower.'
**New coach:** 'Okay, that happened. That choice wasn't the best for me. What is my plan for my next best choice?'

**Old critic:** 'I've completely ruined my progress.'
**New coach:** 'My body is incredibly resilient. One meal doesn't erase weeks of good choices. What's the one thing I can do right now to get back on track?' (Hint: it's the glass of salt water elixir.)

**Old critic:** 'I can't be trusted around food. I'm out of control.'
**New coach:** 'That was a moment of feeling out of control. It's a feeling, not a fact about who I am. What can I take from that moment to help me in the future?' (Maybe you were overtired, or you'd restricted yourself too much the day before.)

Do you see the difference? The old voice is a dead end, a statement of failure. The new voice asks a question. It's a prompt for action. It's forward-looking. It turns a moment of regret into a moment of data collection and strategy.

## YOUR PHYSICAL RESET: THE PATTERN INTERRUPT

Swapping the words in your head is the goal, but sometimes, when you're really in a spiral, it feels like trying to shout over a hurricane. Your brain is stuck in a loop. To break that loop, you need a 'pattern interrupt' – a simple physical action that snaps you out of the trance. When you notice the old, bullying critic starting its monologue, I want you to do one of these two things immediately. It will feel silly at first. That's fine. Just do it anyway.

**Deep breathing reset**

Take four deep breaths: in for four counts, hold for four, out for six. This activates your parasympathetic nervous system and tells your body, 'We're safe.' As you breathe, repeat one of your coaching phrases: 'Okay, that happened. What is my next best choice?'

**The step and reset**

Stand up. Walk out of the room you're in and into a different one. Or, even better, step outside for just 30 seconds. The simple act of changing your physical environment is a powerful signal to your brain to switch it up. As you take a deep breath in your new location, ask the question: 'What's the one thing I can do right now to get back on track?'

These suggestions are grounded in neuroscience. You are using a pattern interrupt to stop a negative neural pathway from firing on autopilot. And in that tiny, precious gap of silence, you can consciously insert your new coaching voice.

## THE SELF-COMPASSION CLAUSE

This all sounds great in theory, but you need a tool for when you're in the thick of it. What happens if you slip up on the reset day itself? You do the morning protocol perfectly, but then at 3 p.m., a colleague offers you a biscuit, and you eat it.

The old critic will immediately scream, 'See? You can't even do the reset day right! You're a total failure!' This is when you invoke a self-compassion clause, by asking the one simple, powerful question the second you realise you've gone off-plan:

'Okay, that happened. What's my next best choice?'

That's it.

You don't spiral. You don't have a go at yourself. You don't scrap the rest of the day. You just acknowledge the blip – the biscuit happened, it's a fact – and you immediately bring your focus to the next decision you have to make. Will your following choice be to have a big glass of water? Will it be to stick to your plan for a Gold Plate dinner? Will it be to go to bed on time?

The reset day isn't about being a perfect robot. It's about practising the skill of getting back on track, over and over again, in real time. Every time you choose to make the *best choice next* instead of spiralling into shame, you are fundamentally rewiring your brain. You are proving to yourself that you are a person who gets back on track, not a person who gives up. That's the real goal here.

## FASTING: WHEN IT HELPS AND WHEN IT DOESN'T

After a big blowout, one of the first things your panicked brain will scream is, 'Right, that's it! I'm not eating today. I'll just fast to make up for it.'

The wellness world is obsessed with fasting. It's presented as a magic bullet for everything from weight loss to longevity. And intermittent fasting can be a useful tool for *some* people, *some* of the time. But using it as a punishment the day after you've eaten the whole pizza? That is a terrible, terrible idea.

Let's get really clear on this.

## WHEN FASTING IS A TERRIBLE IDEA (99 PER CENT OF THE TIME AFTER A BINGE)

You wake up feeling bloated, guilty and your blood sugar is all over the place. Deciding to fast in this state is like trying to put out a fire with a can of petrol. Here's why:

- **It's a punishment, not a strategy:** Let's be honest. You're not doing it for the health benefits. You're doing it because you're angry at yourself. You're using food (or the lack of it) as a way of self-harming. This just strengthens the toxic cycle of bingeing and restricting.
- **It screws up your hormones:** For many women, especially if you're already stressed or in perimenopause, a long fast is just another stressor on your body. It can crank up your stress hormone, cortisol, which can lead to more belly fat storage and even worse cravings later.
- **It sets you up for another binge:** What do you think is going to happen at 4 p.m. after you've had nothing but black coffee all day? You're not going to calmly eat a chicken salad. You are going to become a ravenous goblin who wants to consume the entire contents of the fridge, starting with the carbs. You are creating the problem you're trying to solve.

The day after a blowout, your body does not need deprivation. It needs stability. It needs nutrients. It needs the calm, predictable rhythm of your Gold Plate meals.

## WHEN A 'MINI-FAST' MIGHT BE HELPFUL (THE 1 PER CENT EXCEPTION)

Can adjusting your meal times sometimes help? Yes, but it's not about skipping meals; it's simply about giving your digestion a rest.

- **The scenario:** You had a huge, late dinner. You wake up the next morning and you are genuinely, physically not hungry. You feel stuffed and a bit queasy.
- **The strategy:** You don't need to force-feed yourself your Gold Plate breakfast at 8 a.m. just because it's on the checklist. You can simply listen to your body and wait until you feel genuine hunger signals. This might mean you push your first meal back to 10 or 11 a.m.
- **The crucial difference:** This is not a punishment fast. This is listening to your body. You are waiting for your body's 'I'm ready for fuel' signal. And when that signal comes, you have your full, nourishing Gold Plate meal. You are not skipping a meal; you are just delaying it slightly to honour your body's rhythm.

That's it. For the 24-hour reset, your rule is simple: Don't fast to punish. Eat to stabilise.

> **EATING ON SCHEDULE VS WAITING FOR HUNGER**
>
> There's a difference between 'waiting to feel hungry' as an ideal and 'eating to schedule' as a practical reality. Both are part of this mindset reset journey.
>
> **The reality:** Sometimes you can't wait for perfect hunger signals. If you know you have back-to-back meetings all morning, or a day of travel ahead, you need to eat strategically, not idealistically.

> **Why this matters:** This isn't about not listening to your body — it's about being kind to your future self by preventing a crisis situation. Your body might not be sending hunger signals at 7 a.m., but if you know you won't have another chance to eat until 2 p.m., eating something small and nourishing now is the wise choice.
>
> **The smart move:** Have a small, protein-rich meal or snack during the 30-minute window you DO have. A hard-boiled egg, Greek yogurt, or a protein bar will prevent you from becoming ravenously hungry and reaching for whatever unhealthy options are available later.
>
> **Choose foods that will sustain you rather than just fill a gap:** Protein and healthy fats will keep your blood sugar stable and your energy consistent, even when your day gets chaotic. Think of it as putting fuel in your car before a long journey. You don't wait until you're stranded on the motorway to fill up.
>
> **Side note:** Many clients have told me that by not eating junk carbs for dinner, they have woken up hungry for breakfast ... when did you last feel that? This is what happens when you work with your biology instead of fighting it.

## 24-HOUR HELP

This chapter was your emergency service. You can pull out this plan when you feel like you've gone completely off the rails. Here are the key things to remember.

- **The binge isn't the damage, it's the spiral.** One off-plan meal doesn't ruin anyone's progress. It's the following days of guilt-fuelled punishment or surrender that do the real harm.

- **Use the stop-the-slide protocol.** When you wake up feeling rubbish, your first move is always: one glass of salt water elixir, one gentle walk, and one Gold Plate meal.
- **Follow the 24-hour checklist.** Your only job for the rest of the day is to be kind to your body. Anchor your meals with protein and veg, stay hydrated and get a good night's sleep.
- **Swap your language.** The bully in your head is not your friend. Swap the critical, dead-end statements – e.g. 'I failed' – for calm, action-based questions – e.g. 'What's my next best choice?'
- **Use a pattern interrupt.** If you're stuck in a shame spiral, break the trance. Take some deep, slow breaths or step into a different room. Create a physical gap for your new coaching voice to emerge.
- **Don't fast to punish.** After a blowout, your body needs stability, not starvation. The only time to delay a meal is if you are genuinely, physically not hungry.

## YOUR THIRTEENTH ACTION PLAN: STRATEGIC EATING FOR UNPREDICTABLE SCHEDULES

**The mindset shift:** This isn't about ignoring your hunger signals – you're not betraying intuitive eating; you're practising strategic self-care. Sometimes the most intuitive thing to do is plan ahead. Your body will thank you for the steady energy.

**The goal:** Master the art of eating strategically when your schedule demands it, while still honouring your body's needs and building a sustainable relationship with food.

**The challenge:** You've been taught to 'listen to your body' and eat when hungry, but real life doesn't always cooperate. When you're facing back-to-back meetings, work shifts, travel days or chaotic schedules, waiting for perfect hunger signals can set you up for afternoon crashes and evening binges.

**The practice:** Have 'good to go', healthy sources of food to carry with you at all times.

**In your kitchen:** Keep 5 'strategic snacks' always ready:

- Hard-boiled eggs (batch-cook weekly)
- Individual Greek yogurt pots
- Protein bars you actually like
- Mixed nuts in small containers
- Apple slices with nut butter packets

> **In your work bag:**
> - Emergency protein bar
> - Mixed nuts
> - Protein powder sachet (add to any drink).

We've covered a lot of ground. You have the tools to navigate your hormones, your holidays and even your worst 'I ate the whole pizza' days. You've learned how to be strategic, how to be flexible and how to get back on track with kindness. You have the 'What to do.' You have the 'How to do it.'

But there's one final, crucial piece of the puzzle. It's the thing that makes all this stick. It's the difference between not simply renting these new habits but owning them for life. It's about the story you tell yourself about who you are.

For years, you've probably seen yourself as someone who is 'bad with food', 'always on a diet', or 'just can't stick to anything'.

We've built the skills to disprove that old story. Now, we lock in who you're becoming.

## CHAPTER 14

# THE IDENTITY SHIFT: BECOMING YOU

For the last thirteen chapters, we have been building a toolkit. A seriously impressive one. You learned how to silence the drill sergeant in your head and welcome your new inner coach. You learned how to navigate dieting and exercise myths, sleep challenges and powerful cravings. You have strategies, you have checklists, you have playbooks. You have all the 'what to do' and the 'how to do it'.

But before we go any further, I want to talk about the exhausting and frustrating gap between *knowing* what to do and actually *doing* it. It can feel like having two different people living inside your head.

There's Future You. She's amazing. She's the one you dream about. She gets up early to work out, she meal-preps healthy lunches, she's calm and confident at parties, and she has a fantastic relationship with food. You buy the cute gym clothes and the healthy cookbooks for her. She's the person you know you *could* be. And then there's a knock on the door, and it's Present You. And she's a bit of a mess. She's tired, she's stressed and she just wants to order a takeaway and watch Netflix. She looks at the gym clothes and thinks, 'Maybe tomorrow.' She sees the healthy food in the fridge and thinks, 'That just looks like a lot of effort.'

The story you tell yourself about who you are will always win, and so this final chapter is about that story. It's about ending the internal battle. It's where we stop focusing on the outcomes – your weight, your dress size – and start focusing on the one thing that drives lasting change: your identity.

We are going to focus on the powerful process of *becoming*. Becoming the person who goes for a walk even when she doesn't feel like it. Becoming the person who creates a nourishing meal. Becoming the person who gets back on track the very next day. This is where the habits you've been practising so far start feeling like they are part of who you are. Part of your identity. This is where we lock it in for good. This is where you become the pilot of your life; not just for a day or a week, but for the rest of the flight.

## THE NEW ORDER

Let's acknowledge why every diet you've ever tried has eventually ended in a fiery crash of bingeing and self-loathing. It's because you were taught to build your house from the roof down.

For years, we've all been sold the same three-step plan for change:

- Pick a goal you want to achieve. (The outcome.)
- Figure out a plan to get there. (The process.)
- White-knuckle it with willpower and motivation until you succeed or fail. (The fuel.)

Let's say your goal is to lose a stone for an upcoming holiday (outcome). So you start a punishing diet and workout plan (process). And you try to motivate yourself (fuel). You stick inspirational pictures on the fridge, you tell yourself, 'Nothing tastes as good as skinny feels,' and for a week or two, it might even work.

But you're running on the fumes of excitement. We all know what happens next.

Relying on this type of unrealistic motivation to achieve your goals is like relying on sugar for energy. It gives you an initial rush, but the crash is inevitable and always leaves you worse off than before. As soon as you have a stressful day, a bad night's sleep or just feel a bit fed up, that motivation vanishes. And you're left with a miserable diet and a workout you hate, with no fuel left in the tank.

This is the point where you usually give up. Why? Because the entire process worked against the grain of the most powerful force of all: your *identity*. Deep down, you were trying to follow the actions of a 'super-healthy gym person', while still believing the story that you were 'someone who is bad at diets and hates exercise'. You were trying to change what you *do* without changing who you *are*. It's an unwinnable war.

Okay, so what's the alternative?

We flip the entire thing on its head. The new order, the one that sticks, looks like this: **Identity → Process → Outcome**

Instead of starting with *what you want*, you start with *who you want to be*. This is not some fluffy, 'manifest-it' nonsense. This is a strategic shift that changes the entire game. You stop trying to force yourself into actions that feel unnatural, and instead start taking actions that align with the person you are becoming. Let's break it down.

**The old way (outcome-focused):** 'I want to lose a stone (outcome), so I must force myself to eat this salad and go to the gym (process), even though I hate it and it feels like a punishment.'

**The feeling:** A constant, draining battle against yourself.

**The new way (identity-focused):** 'I am becoming a person who is strong and fuels her body well (identity). Therefore, of course I'm going to have a nourishing lunch and move my body today (process) – that's just what a person like me does. As a result, my body composition will change (outcome).'

**The feeling:** Calm, logical and consistent. Your actions are simply an expression of your identity.

Do you notice the difference? The old way is a punishment. The new way is an identity. In the old model, every healthy choice is a painful reminder of the gap between where you are and where you want to be. In the new model, every healthy choice is a small victory, a little vote that confirms the person you are becoming. We're going to stop trying to willpower our way to an outcome. Instead, we're going to start casting small, daily votes for the identity of the person we want to be. And that is a process that is not only sustainable, but also feels *good*.

Put like this, it almost becomes not about losing weight at all, but simply stepping up to a you that has made the choice to put you first more, to benefit yourself so that you grow quietly stronger, both physically and mentally, by making the right choices. You don't need to decide to change your diet, your behaviour ... you simply need to choose. That's it.

## DEFINING YOUR IDENTITY

So, how do you choose this new identity? We're going to make it incredibly simple. I want you to think of your new identity as a job title. Forget about the outcome for a second. Think about the *feeling* you're chasing. What kind of person experiences that feeling?

- Is it about feeling in control and not letting life's chaos derail you? Maybe your new identity is the Pilot.
- Is it about feeling physically strong, capable and full of life? Maybe you're not just a 'gym-goer', you're the Powerhouse.
- Is it about making intelligent, smart food choices without the drama and deprivation? Maybe you're the Nourisher.

Other ideas to spark your imagination:

- **The Routine Queen** – for the person who wants to build structure and consistency.
- **The Energy Architect** – for the person whose main goal is to build and maintain their energy.
- **The Unshakeable Woman** – for the person who wants to build deep resilience against stress and cravings.

Take 60 seconds right now. Grab a pen. What job title resonates with you? Don't overthink it. What would feel amazing to be? Write it down. This is your new job title. And every action you take from now on is just you showing up for your role.

## HOW TO MAKE DECISIONS

You have decided on your new job title. You are, say, the Powerhouse. But it's 6 a.m., your alarm is screaming, and your bed is warm. How does this new title help you in real life? It becomes your new decision-making filter.

Every choice you make from now on is either a vote for the new person you are, or a vote for the old person you used to be.

That's it. It's that simple.

When the alarm goes off for that walk, you don't ask, 'Do I feel motivated?' You ask, 'What would the Powerhouse do right now?'

The answer is suddenly very simple. She'd get up and go.

- **Hitting the snooze button?** That's a vote for your old self → Getting out of bed and getting dressed? That's a vote for the Routine Queen.
- **Mindlessly grabbing the office biscuit?** It's a vote for your old identity → Pausing and having a glass of water instead? A clear, powerful vote for the Pilot.

This is not about being perfect. This is not about winning every single vote with every choice. This is a democracy, not a dictatorship. You do not need 100 per cent of the votes to win. You just need to win the majority.

Your goal is to cast more votes for your new identity than for your old one each day. When you're faced with a choice, you no longer ask, 'What do I feel like doing?' Instead, you ask a much more powerful question: 'Does this action cast a vote for the woman I am becoming?'

This framework is liberating. It takes the emotion and the white-knuckle drama out of the equation. You're not being 'good' or 'bad'. You are simply casting a vote. And you have the power to cast the next one differently.

## BUILDING YOUR CASE: THE 'EVIDENCE LOG'

Your old identity, someone who quite easily gives up, has a long track record. To help your new identity stick, you need to start collecting evidence. You are now a lawyer constructing a case for your new self. Your job is to collect small, undeniable pieces of proof.

At the end of each day, I want you to open the notes app on your phone and write down one tiny piece of evidence from your day that proves you are becoming your new identity.

- **If you're the Powerhouse:** 'I took the stairs instead of the lift.'
- **If you're the Pilot:** 'I felt a craving coming on, and instead of panicking, I drank a glass of water and paused.'
- **If you're the Nourisher:** 'I added a big handful of spinach to my scrambled eggs this morning.'

These are your tiny 'votes' made real. Every time you write one down, you are stamping it into your brain as proof. After a week, you will have a list of seven pieces of evidence. After a month, you'll have thirty. After a few months, you'll have a mountain of undeniable proof that you *are* this new person. You're not 'faking it till you make it'. You are building your new identity, one tiny, powerful action at a time.

## KEEPING YOUR STREAK ALIVE

You've defined your new identity. You're casting votes for her every day. You're logging your evidence. It feels great.

But then, life happens.

You get slammed with a deadline at work. You get a terrible night's sleep because your neighbour's dog decided 3 a.m. was the perfect time to bark non-stop for an hour. You wake up feeling exhausted, overwhelmed and the idea of doing your usual 45-minute workout feels unrealistic. This is a critical moment. This is where the old you would have said, 'I can't do my full workout, so I'll just do nothing. Today is a write-off.'

But the new you, the identity-focused you, has a much smarter strategy.

## YOUR BARE MINIMUM: THE ANTIDOTE TO ALL-OR-NOTHING

Your bare minimum is that small, almost laughably easy version of your habit that you agree to do on your worst days. It's the version you can do even when you have zero energy, zero time and zero motivation.

The point of this bare minimum is not the physical result. The point of this one is to keep the streak alive and to keep casting a vote for your new identity. Because showing up for five minutes is infinitely more powerful than doing nothing at all.

- **Doing nothing** casts a vote for your old self. It says, 'I'm the kind of person who quits when things get hard.'
- **Doing the bare minimum** casts a vote for your new self. It says, 'I am the kind of person who shows up, even on my worst days.'

The deal? Never miss twice. You might have a day where you're too busy or tired and you do nothing. That's okay. It happens. But you make an agreement with yourself to not let it happen two days in a row. On day two, you show up and you do your bare minimum. Period. This is how you stop one bad day from turning into a bad week.

## YOUR 'EVEN–IF' CONTRACT

This is too important to just think about. Let's make it official. Grab your phone or a piece of paper and write down the answers to these three sentences. This is a contract with your future, overwhelmed self.

- My usual workout habit is _____. On my worst days, my bare minimum is _____. I will do this **even if** I only have 10 minutes.

- My usual nutrition habit is _____. On my worst days, my bare minimum is _____. I will do this **even if** I'm ordering a takeaway.
- My usual self-care habit is _____. On my worst days, my bare minimum is _____. I will do this **even if** I only have 5 minutes before bed.

Look at your answers. This is your emergency plan. It's not a contract to accept failure but to strategically bet on your future self. You've just created a safety net that makes it almost impossible for you to wander off track.

## THE 'WIN THE WEEK' MINDSET

Now, a word of warning. The goal of the chain is not to be a perfect, unbroken, year-long masterpiece. You are a human being with a messy life, not a robot. You will miss a day. The chain will break. And that is okay. Your new goal is to win the week. At the end of the week, look at your calendar. If you see more ticks than blank spaces, you have won. If you completed four days, it's a win. Five is a landslide victory. In a truly horrendous week, even a one is a win, because you showed up once when you could've shown up zero times.

This mindset kills perfectionism. It allows for life with all its ups and downs. You're not aiming for an unblemished record; you're aiming to be a person who, more often than not, shows up for herself.

## HOW TO RECOVER FAST: CHAIN REACTIONS

Let's imagine you break the chain of ticks. You have a terrible weekend, you do nothing, and now it's Monday morning. The guilt is heavy, and it feels like you've lost all momentum. The old you would look at the mountain of 'perfect choices' you need to make to get back on track and feel completely overwhelmed. The new you understands that you don't need to climb the whole mountain at once. Your only job is to follow the stop-the-slide protocol.

Remember, make your first good choice and you'll start a positive chain reaction.

Drink one glass of water.

Go for one walk.

Prepare one Gold Plate.

When you feel lost, stop looking at the mountain. Just start with the first step back into the game. Once you've taken that step, you can start your next chain of ticks on your calendar. See? You're winning again.

## THE 10-DAY UNBREAKABLE CHALLENGE

This challenge has one purpose and one purpose only: to build a moutain of undeniable proof that you are the person you've decided to become. This is about proving to yourself, with ten consecutive days of action, that you are a woman who shows up for herself.

Let me be crystal clear about what this is not. This is not a '10-day shred'. This is not about losing weight, getting a flat stomach or detoxing. I couldn't care less what the bathroom scales say at the end of it.

This is the 'unbreakable' challenge for a reason. Because with the bare minimum rule as your safety net, it is almost impossible to fail.

### THE BIG IDEA

For the next 10 days, your only goal is to show up and complete five simple actions every single day. We'll call them your 'Daily 5.'

Ten days is short enough to not feel overwhelming, but long enough to build real momentum and create a powerful streak. Think of this challenge as your 10-day job orientation for your new role as the Powerhouse identity or the Routine Queen. The 'Daily 5' are not just random tasks; they are your job's core duties.

## *Your Daily 5*
1. Follow your Gold Plate formula
2. Mixed movement
3. The hydration protocol
4. Practise your power-down hour
5. The identity shift

These aren't random tasks; they're the habits that reinforce everything you've learned.

And so, these five actions are your non-negotiables for the next 10 days. Remember, your **bare minimum** for each of these absolutely counts as a win.

1. **The Gold Plate** builds stable energy and stops the craving cycle. Your mission is to have at least one 'Gold Plate' meal each day. Just one. That's a meal anchored with protein, veggies and healthy fats. (Your bare minimum might be just making sure one meal has a solid source of protein.)
2. **Movement:** Strength training is your metabolic pension and confidence builder. Your mission is to complete one strength session (even if it's just 20 minutes using your emergency protocols). For your LISS movement it's a brisk walk. (Your bare minimum might be 10 push-ups and a 10-minute walk.)
3. **Salt water elixir:** Carry your water bottle and sip regularly rather than chugging massive amounts. (Your bare minimum

might be just that morning salt water elixir and one extra glass of water.)
4. **The power-down hour** protects your recovery and hormone balance. Your mission is to have a 'digital sunset' one hour before you plan to sleep. All screens off. Phone, laptop, TV. Give your brain a chance to power down. (Your bare minimum might be just putting your phone on the other side of the room 15 minutes before bed.)
5. **Progress tracking** builds evidence of your new identity. Your mission is to write down one piece of evidence that proves you are your new identity. Not calories, just completion. (Your bare minimum can be one tiny vote you cast for yourself, such as 'I took the stairs' or 'I drank water instead of diet cola.')

Before you begin the challenge, copy these five actions into your notebook. This simple act turns a to-do list into an identity-building mission: 'I am someone who nourishes her body, builds her strength and shows up consistently.'

## *The unbreakable scorecard*

This is not a test; it's a scorecard. Grab a notebook or a piece of paper and draw this simple grid.

|  | Day 1 | Day 2 | Day 3 | Day 4 | Day 5 | Day 6 | Day 7 | Day 8 | Day 9 | Day 10 |
|---|---|---|---|---|---|---|---|---|---|---|
| 1. Gold Plate |  |  |  |  |  |  |  |  |  |  |
| 2. Move for 20 |  |  |  |  |  |  |  |  |  |  |
| 3. Hydrate Smart |  |  |  |  |  |  |  |  |  |  |
| 4. Log Evidence |  |  |  |  |  |  |  |  |  |  |
| 5. Digital Sunset |  |  |  |  |  |  |  |  |  |  |

At the end of each day, you give yourself a simple tick (✓) for each of the 'Daily 5' you completed. Remember, doing your bare minimum gets you a full tick! After 10 days, you will have a scorecard with up to 50 ticks on it. That is 50 pieces of undeniable proof; 50 votes you have cast for the woman you are becoming. You will have a 10-day streak of showing up for yourself.

This is about identity. This is your launchpad. This is where you stop hoping that you can *change* and start proving to yourself that you already *are*.

## HOW TO TAME YOUR GREMLINS: YOUR 10-DAY TROUBLESHOOTING GUIDE

Over the 10 days, the little gremlin in your head – the voice of your old self – is going to pop up with some very predictable complaints. Here's what it will say, and next to it is your new, calm, identity-based response.

*Gremlin complaint 1: 'I'm too tired to move today.'*
**Your new response:** 'Okay, I hear that. And an Energy Architect knows that a short 10-minute walk will actually *create* energy, not spend it. Let's do the bare minimum.'

*Gremlin complaint 2: 'I deserve a treat. One day off won't hurt.'*
**Your new response:** 'You're right, this isn't about punishment. But what I deserve even more is the feeling of keeping a promise to myself. A Routine Queen knows that consistency is the ultimate reward. Let me find a way to have a treat that still aligns with my goals.'

*Gremlin complaint 3: 'This is pointless. It's not making a difference fast enough.'*
**Your new response:** 'This isn't about the outcome; it's about the identity. The goal today isn't to lose weight; it's to cast a vote. A

Powerhouse knows that strength is built one rep at a time. I'm just doing my reps, however few they are.'

**Gremlin complaint 4 (after a slip-up): 'See? You've messed it up. Might as well quit.'**
**Your new response:** 'This is not a pass-or-fail test. This is an experiment. The Pilot knows that turbulence is normal. My only job is to get back on course with my very next action.'

Read these over. Know that these thoughts will come. And now, you have a plan for them. You're not just ready for the actions, you're ready for the resistance.

# YOUR FOURTEENTH ACTION PLAN: TRACKING YOUR STREAKS

**The mindset shift:** If you've just had a 'blowout' meal or day, your only job is to make your very next meal a good one. Not tomorrow, not Monday – your next meal. One good choice erases the drama and gets you straight back on track.

**The goal:** Your brain loves to win. It loves seeing visual proof of progress. So, we're going to make this a game: Don't Break The Chain.

**The task:** Get a calendar. One of those big, physical wall calendars. Every day you succeed in casting a vote for your new identity, whether that's following your system properly or just your bare minimum, you get to draw a big, satisfying tick through that date. Your only goal is to not break the chain of ticks.

**The practice:** Crossing out the days will motivate you to keep going. After you've got a chain of five, ten, twenty ticks in a row, you will find it much harder to skip a day. You won't want to break that beautiful chain you've built. That chain is a visual representation of your new identity. It's proof that you are the person who shows up.

# MILESTONE 3: THE 12-WEEK CHALLENGE

Okay, you've just had a crash course in changing your mindset around food and dieting. You're on a roll. You have a bank of new knowledge, and you're feeling like a total rockstar. And, right on cue, that familiar, nagging voice pipes up in the back of your head: 'This is great ... but how long can you actually keep this up? How do you do this forever?'

The thought of being 'perfect' every single day for the rest of your life is enough to make you want to lie down and never get up from your sofa. It sounds exhausting. It sounds impossible. And honestly? That would be.

This is the point where we need to have a serious chat about the difference between a sprint and a cruise. Your old all-or-nothing self only had two speeds: a full-on, desperate sprint, or stationary. There was no in between. You couldn't maintain the sprint, so you crashed out.

The new you understands that you can't sprint forever. You need those seasons. You need a rhythm.

It can be helpful to break down your year into blocks of time to make it easier to follow the plan. It can help you stay in the game for the long haul and maintain your forever body.

Try this new rhythm for life:

>12-week sprint → 4-week cruise →
>12-week sprint → 4-week cruise

You will deliberately cycle between periods of high focus and periods of relaxed maintenance.

This pattern is the ultimate antidote to burnout. It honours the fact that you can't be perfectly 'on it' 365 days a year. It gives you permission to have seasons of intense effort and seasons of ease, all while moving you consistently in the right direction.

Remember, this is not a diet. It's your personal operating system for a lifetime of progress and your forever body.

## THE 12-WEEK SPRINT: YOUR SEASON OF FOCUS

Think in roughly 12-week cycles. A 12-week block is your sprint phase. It's a season of intentional focus and growth where you are actively pushing for progress. It's where you turn up the dial on your focus and effort to an 8 or 9 out of 10.

**During a sprint:** You're committed with your choices, consistent with your workouts and probably logging your progress daily. A 12-week sprint is long enough to see incredible results but short enough that it has a clear finish line, which stops it from feeling like a life sentence.

## THE 4-WEEK CRUISE PHASE: THE ART OF EFFORTLESS MAINTENANCE

At the end of your 12-week sprint, you don't stop. You simply shift gears into 'cruise'. This is your maintenance season. It's where you reap the rewards of your hard work and practise living with your new habits in a more relaxed way. It's not about pushing forward; it's simply about not slipping back. You turn the dial down to a comfortable 5 or 6 and simply live within your new, upgraded normal.

**During a cruise:** The non-negotiables of your identity remain but the rules become more flexible. You use your intuition more and your rulebook a little less. The goal is to hold your ground, enjoy your life and maintain your progress.

## YOUR 'CRUISE CONTROL' PERMISSION SLIP

Let's be honest, the idea of the cruise phase might feel a bit scary. The little voice in your head might be whispering, 'But won't I just slide all the way back? Isn't this just a slippery slope back to my old habits?' That's the old you talking. The cruise phase is not about letting go of the wheel. It's about taking your foot off the accelerator and setting the cruise control. You are still heading in the right direction; you're just using less energy to do it.

Here is your permission slip for this phase.

- **You have permission to trust your new identity.** You spent 12 weeks building the habits of the new you. You don't need to micromanage her anymore. She knows how to prepare a good meal. Trust that.
- **You have permission for your data to get 'fuzzier'.** You don't need to log every single thing. Your new job is to focus on the big data: Am I generally getting my protein in? Am I moving my body a few times a week? Am I getting enough sleep?
- **You have permission to regain a little.** Sometimes, in a sprint, we are a little dehydrated or depleted. The cruise phase is where your body finds its happy, sustainable settling point. This is not failure; it's equilibrium.

## THE FINISH LINE: YOUR BEFORE AND AFTER REFLECTION

You did it. You have completed your first full sprint. *Well done.*

Before you read another word, I want you to just stop. Close your eyes. I want you to think back, really think back, to the woman who started this journey. Picture her. Think about her fears, her frustrations, and the quiet, flickering hope she was holding on to.

You've kept that hope alive. You'll have shown up for her, day after day, vote by vote. You should be incredibly, profoundly proud of yourself. This isn't just the end of a plan; it's a moment to truly acknowledge the distance you have travelled. It's time to create the most honest and powerful 'before and after' picture you will ever have – one that has nothing to do with the number on a set of scales.

## YOUR WEEKEND MISSION

This isn't a test. This is a quiet, personal ceremony. Find an hour for yourself, make your favourite drink, and create a space to reflect on your journey.

### PART 1: THE BEFORE AND AFTER SNAPSHOT

It's time to take a snapshot of who you were before we began this journey together and who you've become today. On a fresh page in your notebook or in your notes on your phone, answer these three simple questions.

- **What is the one word that describes how I felt *before*?** (e.g. 'Stuck', 'chaotic', 'tired'.)
- **What is the one word that describes how I feel *now*?** (e.g. 'Strong', 'calm', 'capable'.)

- **What are the two or three non-negotiable habits that are now just a part of who I am?** (e.g. '1. Protein at breakfast. 2. Two strength workouts a week.')

Now let these statements sit. Absorb them. Acknowledge their worth and reflect on how far you've come since we started. You have fundamentally changed the way you feel about yourself by habit-stacking week after week. You've worked hard and we should mark this milestone.

## PART 2: THE FIRST TASTE OF 'FOREVER AFTER'

Your final task is to plan your first act of celebration to raise up the person you have become – a person who can navigate life with skill, not restriction.

Plan something for the week ahead that has nothing to do with rules and everything to do with joy, handled with your new, confident mindset. Perhaps book a table at that restaurant you love and use your 'pick two' playbook with ease; buy that outfit you've been eyeing, not because you've hit a goal, but because you feel good in your own skin *right now*; or plan a weekend day with zero obligations, purely for rest, and protect that time fiercely.

## CHAPTER 15
# THE ONLY MINDSET YOU NEED

This is it. You've held a conversation with your past self and made a plan for your future self. You see the change not in numbers, but in feelings and in habits. You are not on a diet. You are not on a plan. You are simply a woman who knows, deep in her bones, how to take incredible care of herself.

Here is your new operating system in a nutshell.

- **Identity over everything.** Stop trying to get motivated. Start deciding who you want to become. Your actions will follow your identity.
- **Every choice is a vote.** You are either casting a vote for the woman you want to become or the woman you used to be. Your only job is to win most of the votes each day, not every single one.
- **Use your bare minimum.** On your worst days, showing up for five minutes is an infinite win over doing nothing. It keeps your identity streak alive. Your new rule is: never miss twice.
- **Win the week, don't be perfect.** The goal is not an unbroken chain of perfection. If you have more winning days than losing days, you are winning at life.

- **Recover fast.** When you fall off track, your only job is to find the one tiny action that starts the positive chain reaction again. Drink one glass of salt water elixir. Go for one 10-minute walk.
- **Sprint and cruise.** You can't be 'on it' constantly. Use the focused 12-week sprints to make progress and relaxed 4-week cruises to maintain it. This is how you avoid burnout for good.
- **Anchor it all to your North Star.** When you connect your daily actions to a deep value, like 'freedom' or 'strength', your fuel becomes infinite.

## YOUR MENTAL TOOLKIT: THE GREMLIN-TAMING GUIDE

This is your 'in case of emergency' helpline. When you're in a panic, you need powerful tools close by.

### When you feel an intense craving, use:

- **The craving decision sequence:** 1. Drink a full glass of water. 2. Pause for 5 minutes. 3. If craving remains, have a protein anchor. 4. If it *still* remains, use the 15-minute rule and a stress script (see pages 213 and 215).

### When you're in a shame spiral, use:

- **The pattern interrupt:** Take some long, slow breaths or step into a different room to break the trance.
- **The critic vs coach language swap:** Replace 'I failed' with, 'Okay, that happened. What's my next best choice?'

### When you have a slip-up (even on a reset day), use:

- **The self-compassion clause:** Set a 5-minute timer and do one small thing that moves you forward – no overthinking allowed.

### When you're facing a tough choice, use:

- **Do a North Star check:** Ask yourself: 1. 'Does this move me closer to my North Star?' 2. 'Which choice will future me be happier that I made?'

Remember that North Star we talked about at the very beginning of the book (page 9)? That deeper reason you picked up this book – not to achieve a dress size or a number on the bathroom scales, but to become the woman you wanted to become?

Every tool in this book has been quietly guiding you towards her. The Gold Plate wasn't really about perfect nutrition – it was about becoming someone who nourishes herself consistently; the 40-minute workouts weren't about burning calories – they were about building evidence that you're someone who shows up for herself; the reset protocols weren't about damage control – they were about proving you're someone who treats herself with compassion, even after difficult moments.

Your North Star was never about the food or the exercise. It was about becoming the woman who moves through the world with quiet confidence. The woman who has made peace with her body. The woman who can trust herself around any food, in any situation. The woman who models genuine self-care for everyone in her life.

That woman isn't some future version of yourself that you'll become when you 'reach your goal'. She's been emerging with every choice you've made along this journey: every time you chose the salad not because you had to, but because you wanted to fuel yourself well; every time you completed a workout not to punish yesterday's choices, but to honour your body's strength; every time you practised the reset protocol not from a place of shame, but from a place of love.

You've been living as her all along.

The beautiful truth is that your North Star isn't a destination – it's a way of being. It's not something you achieve once and then maintain forever. It's something you choose, again and again, in countless small moments throughout your days.

## FROM VALUES TO BEHAVIOURS: YOUR UNBREAKABLE CHAIN

Values are the big, powerful words that describe what truly matters to you deep down; they are what is your driving force. They are the fundamental beliefs that shape you. Things like:

- **HEALTH:** Not just the absence of sickness, but your core sense of wellbeing, energy and quality of life.
- **FREEDOM:** Freedom from food obsession, from hiding in photos, from feeling limited by your body.
- **STRENGTH:** The physical and mental resilience to handle whatever life throws at you.
- **PRESENCE:** The ability to be fully engaged with your kids, your partner and your life, not stuck in your head worrying about food or your body.

A goal is temporary, but a value is permanent. And when you connect your daily actions to a core value, they stop being chores and start being sacred.

This is how this unbreakable chain works:

Your VALUE (the North Star) →
Your IDENTITY (the person you are) →
Your BEHAVIOUR (the vote you cast)

Let's see it in action:

### *Your North Star Value is FREEDOM*
- The **identity** you chose to live out that value was the (e.g.) Pilot.
- When you're faced with a craving, the **behaviour** of pausing and drinking a glass of water isn't a diet rule. It's a vote for **FREEDOM** from being hijacked by your urges.

### *Your North Star Value is STRENGTH*
- The **identity** you chose was the (e.g.) Powerhouse.
- The **behaviour** of going to the gym when you're tired isn't a punishment. It's a vote for **STRENGTH**.

### *Your North Star Value is PRESENCE*
- The **identity** you chose was the (e.g.) Nourisher.
- The behaviour of building a Gold Plate meal isn't about restriction. It's a vote for having the stable energy you need to be fully **PRESENT** with your family tonight.

Do you feel that? That your tiny, daily actions are the physical manifestation of your deepest values. What matters is how you *live*.

There will, of course, still be challenging moments ahead. Days when the old patterns call to you. Times when motivation feels distant and the path feels unclear. In those moments, you don't need to remember every strategy in this book. You just need to remember your North Star. Ask yourself: 'What would the woman I'm becoming choose right now?'

The answer will always guide you home.

You are not on a diet. You are not following a plan. You are simply a woman who knows, deep in her bones, how to take incredible care of herself. You are someone who understands that true strength isn't about perfection – it's about showing up, especially when it's hard.

Welcome to your forever after.

# AFTERWORD
## FINAL LETTER TO FUTURE YOU

Before we finish, I want you to do one last thing for me. I want you to write a letter. But it's not to me. It's to the woman you'll be in a year's time. To the woman who has been living as the Powerhouse or the Pilot, and owning it completely, through multiple cycles. She's completed the sprint, the cruise; she's faced the challenge of giving up but has carried on day after day.

This letter will be a time capsule. It's a snapshot of your 'why', your powerful North Star. Writing it will be the ultimate act of self-affirmation, committing your new identity and habits to paper so that you can honour them forever.

## STEP 1: WRITING PROMPTS

Grab a piece of paper or open a new note on your phone. Don't worry about writing a perfect letter; just answer these questions from the heart. Let the words be messy and honest.

- **Start by describing today.** Where are you sitting? How do you feel in your body and your mind *right now*, having completed your first sprint cycle? (e.g. 'I feel confident and proud that I've reached the end of my first 12 weeks of the plan ...'
- **What is one feeling you experienced at the beginning of your 12-week journey?** Name it. Was it the feeling of being out of

control? Of shame? Of constant exhaustion? (e.g. 'I was so tired of feeling weak and disappointed in myself every evening ...')

- **What is the one feeling you have been most excited to welcome in?** This is your North Star. (e.g. 'I was so excited to feel that sense of FREEDOM in my own skin ...')
- **What was your biggest fear about this journey?** Be honest. (e.g. 'I was scared I would be the same person after 12 weeks, and that this would be another thing I've failed at ...')
- **Give her one piece of advice for the future.** What is the one thing you want to remind her of if she's having a tough day? (e.g. 'Please remember that it was never about being perfect. Just remember to be kind and start again with the next choice ...')
- **Finally, ask her a question.** What is the one thing you are most curious to know about her life? (e.g. 'I have to know ... are you finally sleeping through the night?')

I want you to talk to her. Tell her what you're hoping for. Tell her what you're a bit scared of. Tell her what you're most excited about.

Maybe you'll write something like:

*Dear Future Me,*

*I'm writing this from the sofa on a Tuesday night. I'm at the end of my first 12-week sprint. Before, I was tired of the all-or-nothing cycle. I was tired of feeling at war with my own body. I guess I was a bit scared I would fail at this, just like I have in the past.*

*But I'm also hopeful now I've completed my first 12 weeks. I'm excited about the idea of not thinking about food all the time. I'm excited about feeling strong in my body, not just slimmer. I'm hoping you feel that, too. I hope you feel the FREEDOM we talked about.*

*I hope you've been kind to yourself. I hope you remembered that it's not about being perfect, but about just showing up. I hope you're proud of all the small votes you've cast for yourself, day after day.*

*I can't wait to see you and look at how far you've come in a year.*

## STEP 2: THE CEREMONY: SEAL IT AND LET IT GO

When you've finished writing, I want you to treat this letter with the respect it deserves. This isn't just a note: it's a contract with your future self.

- **If you've written it on paper:** Fold it, put it in an envelope, and write on the front: '**To be opened on [date one year from today].**' Then, put it somewhere you won't be tempted to open it, but where you won't forget it.
- **If you've written it on your phone/computer:** This is even more powerful. Search online for 'email to future self' services – there are several free websites that allow you to write an email and schedule it to be delivered to your inbox at a future date of your choosing. Simply copy and paste your letter, set the delivery date for one year from now, and send it to yourself. You'll receive your own words exactly when you need to hear them most.

The act of physically sealing the letter or digitally sending it into the future is crucial. It is an act of trust. You are letting go of the person you were 12 weeks before and making space for the person you are becoming. You are trusting that she is here and will be in a year's time, too.

In a year from now, that letter will land in your inbox or in your hands. It will be a message from a woman you could only dream of, reminding you just how far you've come.

I am so incredibly proud of the woman who is taking the time to write this letter today; of her courage, for her hope and for her decision to finally, truly show up for herself. And I am so excited for the woman who will one day read it.

You've got this. All of it. Now, go and become her.

# REFERENCE SECTION

I've put a lot of the tables and lists here, as an easier way to find them for reference.

## 1. THE 2-WEEK MIX-AND-MATCH MEAL PLANNER

Pick one option from each category per day. For dinners, you can cook a double portion to have for lunch the next day (smart leftovers!).

### Breakfasts (choose 1)

- **The 3-minute scramble:** 2–3 eggs scrambled in butter or olive oil with a huge handful of spinach and a sprinkle of feta.
- **The power bowl:** A big bowl of full-fat Greek yogurt, a scoop of your favourite protein powder, a handful of berries and a sprinkle of almonds.
- **The quick smoothie:** 1 scoop protein powder, a handful of spinach, ½ banana, 1 tbsp nut butter and unsweetened almond milk or water.
- **The savoury start:** A bowl of cottage cheese with sliced tomatoes, cucumber, salt, pepper and a drizzle of olive oil.

### Lunches (choose 1)

- **The giant salad:** A huge bed of mixed greens, a palm-sized portion of protein (tinned tuna, leftover chicken, chickpeas), lots of colourful veg and a simple olive oil and lemon juice dressing.
- **The smart leftovers:** A portion of last night's dinner. The easiest and best lunch there is.
- **The deconstructed burrito bowl:** A base of mixed greens topped with a scoop of salsa, a scoop of guacamole, black beans and your choice of leftover protein.

### Dinners (choose 1)

- **Simple salmon and greens:** A salmon fillet baked or pan-fried, served with a mountain of roasted broccoli or asparagus tossed in olive oil.
- **Chicken stir-fry:** Chicken breast stir-fried with a ton of colourful peppers, onions and snap peas in a simple soy-ginger sauce. Serve as is, or with a small portion of brown rice.
- **Turkey mince chilli:** Turkey mince cooked with kidney beans, chopped tomatoes and spices. Serve over a bed of lettuce and top with a dollop of Greek yogurt and avocado.
- **The better burger:** A good-quality beef or turkey burger (no bun) served with a huge side salad and a few sweet potato wedges.

### Snacks (have 1 to 2, only if genuinely hungry)

- An apple with a spoonful of peanut butter.
- A handful of almonds.
- A hard-boiled egg.
- A small pot of full-fat Greek yogurt.

## 2. THE MOVEMENT MENU: YOUR NO-NONSENSE WORKOUT PLAN

Remember the philosophy: this is about building strength, not punishment. Your bare minimum is always a win.

### *Your movement plan: 2–3 times a week*

Alternate between Workout A and Workout B on non-consecutive days (e.g. Monday: A; Wednesday: B; Friday: A; and so on). Aim for 3 sets of 8 to 12 reps for each exercise. Choose a weight that feels more challenging for the last two reps.

### *Workout A: Full body*

- **Goblet squats:** Hold one dumbbell vertically against your chest and squat down as if sitting in a chair. Keep your chest up.
- **Push-ups:** On your toes or on your knees. Lower your chest towards the floor and push back up.
- **Dumbbell rows:** Lean on a bench with one knee and one hand. Hold a dumbbell in the other hand and pull it up towards your hip, squeezing your back.
- **Glute bridges:** Lie on your back with your knees bent. Place a dumbbell across your hips and drive your hips up towards the ceiling.
- **Plank:** Hold a straight line from your head to your heels. Aim for 30 to 60 seconds.

### *Workout B: Full body*

- **Dumbbell deadlifts:** Hold a dumbbell in each hand in front of your thighs. Keeping your legs almost straight, hinge at your hips and lower the weights towards the floor. Squeeze your bum to stand back up.
- **Overhead press:** Sit or stand, holding a dumbbell in each hand at shoulder height. Press the weights directly overhead.

- **Reverse lunges:** Step one foot back and lower both knees to a 90-degree angle. Push off the back foot to return to standing. Using dumbbells is optional.
- **Glute kickbacks:** On all fours, bend your leg and kick one leg back and up, squeezing your glute. Add a dumbbell behind the knee for an extra challenge.
- **Leg raises:** Lie on your back and slowly lower your straight legs towards the floor without letting your lower back arch. Important: Everyone's range of motion is different – stop lowering your legs the moment you feel your lower back start to lift off the floor or arch. This is your safe range, and it will improve over time. Never force your legs lower than your body can handle while maintaining proper form.

## 3. COOKING WITH HAND MEASURES

Choose one item from at least three of the four columns below to create your perfect meal. This is your ultimate cheat sheet for an optimal meal, every single time.

| 1. Pick your protein (1 palm) | 2. Load up on fibre (2 fists) | 3. Add your smart carbs (1 cupped hand) | 4. Don't forget healthy fats (1 thumb) | 5. Gut health boosters (optional sprinkle) |
|---|---|---|---|---|
| PRO TIP: Choose the best quality you can afford – organic, grass-fed or free-range when possible. Your body will use high-quality protein more efficiently. | PRO TIP: Vegetables with the ® symbol are tastiest roasted at 200°C/400°F with olive oil and salt, until tender. | PRO TIP: Cook and cool starches like potatoes and rice to increase their gut-friendly resistant starch. | PRO TIP: Prioritise omega-3 fats (marked with an *) for their anti-inflammatory power. | PRO TIP: A tablespoon or two is all you need to support your gut microbiome. |

## REFERENCE SECTION

| 1. Pick your protein (1 palm) | 2. Load up on fibre (2 fists) | 3. Add your smart carbs (1 cupped hand) | 4. Don't forget healthy fats (1 thumb) | 5. Gut health boosters (optional sprinkle) |
|---|---|---|---|---|
| POULTRY | LEAFY GREENS | STARCHY and ROOT VEG | OILS and DRESSINGS | FERMENTED FOODS |
| Turkey mince or escalope | Spinach (raw or wilted) | Sweet potato ® | Extra-virgin olive oil | Kimchi |
| Chicken breasts or thighs | Rocket | New potatoes (boiled) ® | Avocado oil | Unsweetened kefir |
| FISH and SEAFOOD | Kale (drizzled with oil) ® | Butternut squash ® | Flaxseed oil* | Miso (in soups / dressings) |
| Salmon fillet* | Lettuce (all types) | Carrots ® | Vinaigrette (oil-based) | Apple cider vinegar |
| Cod, hake, pollock or haddock fillet | | Parsnips ® | | Sauerkraut |
| Tinned tuna in oil / water | CRUCIFEROUS POWERHOUSES | | NUTS and SEEDS | Kombucha |
| Sardines* / mackerel* | Broccoli (cut into florets) ® | GRAINS and LEGUMES | Almonds / walnuts* | |
| Prawns / shrimp | Cauliflower (cut into florets) ® | Quinoa (pre-cooked is great) | Pistachios / Brazil nuts | |
| RED MEAT | Brussels sprouts (halved) ® | Brown or wild rice | Chia seeds* / flaxseeds* | |
| Lamb (chops, minced) | Cabbage (thinly sliced) ® | Lentils (all colours) | Hemp seeds* / pumpkin seeds | |
| Lean beef mince | COLOURFUL FAVOURITES | Chickpeas | Tahini | |
| Steak (sirloin, flank) | Green beans (topped and tailed) | Black beans / kidney beans | | |

| 1. Pick your protein (1 palm) | 2. Load up on fibre (2 fists) | 3. Add your smart carbs (1 cupped hand) | 4. Don't forget healthy fats (1 thumb) | 5. Gut health boosters (optional sprinkle) |
|---|---|---|---|---|
| DAIRY and PLANT-BASED | Peppers (deseeded, sliced) ® | | WHOLE FOODS This section is for minimally processed foods or specify 'homemade versions' where applicable. | |
| Lentils / beans | Asparagus (snap off woody ends) ® | FRUITS | Avocado | |
| Cottage cheese | Courgette (sliced) | Berries (all types) | Olives | |
| Eggs (4) | Aubergine (cubed) ® | Apple or pear | Homemade pesto (check for good oils) | |
| Tofu or tempeh (firm) | Mushrooms (sliced) | Banana | Dark chocolate (70 per cent+ cocoa) | |
| Greek yogurt (full-fat) | Onions (sliced) ® | Orange or peach | Brewer's yeast | |
| | Tomatoes (all types) ® | Mango, pineapple, grapes, kiwi, melon, etc. | | |

- **Pick your protein:** You have some frozen salmon fillets. Perfect. Bake one (1 palm).
- **Load up on veggies:** There's a head of broccoli and a bag of spinach. Chop the broccoli into florets to roast or steam (1 fist) and wilt the spinach (1 fist) at the last minute.
- **Add your smart carbs:** A pouch of pre-cooked quinoa is at the back of the cupboard. Easiest decision ever. Heat some up (1 cupped hand).

- **Don't forget healthy fats:** Use olive oil to roast the broccoli, or drizzle it on the salmon (1 thumb).
- **Gut health booster (optional):** Add a tablespoon of kimchi on the side for some spicy, gut-friendly goodness.

## 4. RECIPE CARDS USING PREPPED BASES

### Recipe card 1: chicken power bowl

**Prep time:** 5 minutes

1. Place 1 cupped hand of quinoa in a bowl.
2. Top with 1 palm portion of sliced chicken.
3. Add 1 fist of roasted vegetables.
4. Make dressing: 1 tbsp olive oil + 1 tbsp lemon juice + pinch of salt.
5. Add a large handful of fresh spinach.
6. Drizzle dressing over everything.
7. Sprinkle with 1 tbsp pine nuts or almonds.

**Why this works:** Complete protein + complex carbs + healthy fats + fibre + antioxidants

### Recipe card 2: chicken and veggie stir-fry

**Prep time:** 10 minutes

1. Heat 1 tsp olive oil in a pan.
2. Add 1 palm portion of pre-cooked chicken (warm through for 2 minutes).
3. Add 1 fist of roasted vegetables (warm for 2 minutes).
4. Make sauce: 2 tbsp soy sauce + 1 tsp fresh grated ginger.
5. Pour sauce over chicken and vegetables.
6. Serve over 1 cupped hand of quinoa.
7. Top with handful of fresh spinach and 1 tbsp chopped almonds.

**Why this works:** Anti-inflammatory ginger + complete amino acids + sustained energy

### Recipe card 3: pesto chicken quinoa salad
**Prep time:** 5 minutes
1. Let pre-cooked quinoa come to room temperature.
2. Mix 1 cupped hand quinoa with 2 tbsp good-quality pesto.
3. Add 1 palm portion of diced chicken.
4. Mix in 1 fist of roasted vegetables (chopped smaller).
5. Add a large handful of rocket or spinach.
6. Drizzle with 1 tsp extra olive oil.
7. Top with 1 tbsp walnuts and cherry tomatoes.

**Why this works:** Brain-healthy omega-3s + sustained energy + gut-friendly fibre

### Recipe card 4: chicken and hummus wrap
**Prep time:** 5 minutes
1. Take 1 large wholemeal tortilla.
2. Spread 3 tbsp hummus across the wrap.
3. Add 1 palm portion of sliced chicken.
4. Add 1 fist of roasted vegetables.
5. Add a handful of fresh spinach or lettuce.
6. Squeeze fresh lemon juice over filling.
7. Drizzle with 1 tsp olive oil.
8. Roll tightly and slice in half.

**Why this works:** Portable + protein + fibre + healthy fats + blood sugar balance

### Recipe card 5: warming chicken and vegetable quinoa bowl
**Prep time:** 10 minutes
1. Heat 1 tsp olive oil in a pan.

2. Add 1 cupped hand quinoa with 2 tbsp water (warm for 2 minutes).
3. Add 1 palm portion chicken and 1 fist vegetables (warm through).
4. Season with salt, pepper and 1 tsp ground turmeric.
5. Transfer to a bowl and add handful of fresh spinach (will wilt).
6. Drizzle with 1 tbsp olive oil mixed with lemon juice.
7. Top with 1 tbsp pumpkin seeds.

**Why this works:** Anti-inflammatory turmeric + warming + hormone-supporting healthy fats

### *Recipe card 6: Greek-style chicken salad*

**Prep Time:** 5 minutes

1. Create salad base with large handful of spinach and rocket.
2. Add 1 cupped hand of quinoa.
3. Top with 1 palm portion of chicken.
4. Add 1 fist of roasted vegetables.
5. Make Greek dressing: 1 tbsp olive oil + 1 tsp red wine vinegar + pinch of dried oregano.
6. Add 5 to 6 olives and 1 tbsp crumbled feta cheese.
7. Drizzle dressing over everything.

**Why this works:** Mediterranean diet benefits + probiotics from cheese + antioxidant-rich olives

### *Recipe card 7: protein-packed quinoa 'fried rice'*

**Prep time:** 10 minutes

1. Heat 1 tsp olive oil in a large pan.
2. Add 1 cupped hand quinoa (fry for 2 minutes until slightly crispy).
3. Push quinoa to one side, scramble 1 egg in the empty space.
4. Mix egg through quinoa.

5. Add 1 palm portion diced chicken and 1 fist vegetables.
6. Season with 2 tbsp soy sauce + 1 tsp sesame oil.
7. Top with handful of fresh spinach and 1 tbsp sesame seeds.

**Why this works:** Extra protein from egg + satisfying texture + B vitamins for energy

### Recipe card 8: Mediterranean stuffed sweet potato

**Prep Time:** 5 minutes (if you have pre-baked sweet potato)
1. Take 1 medium baked sweet potato, slice open.
2. Fluff flesh with a fork.
3. Top with 1 palm portion of warm chicken.
4. Add 1 fist of roasted vegetables.
5. Make tahini dressing: 1 tbsp tahini + 1 tsp lemon juice + 1 tsp water.
6. Add handful of fresh spinach.
7. Drizzle with tahini dressing.
8. Sprinkle with 1 tbsp chopped almonds.

**Why this works:** Beta-carotene + complete protein + healthy fats + satisfying comfort food feel

### Recipe card 9: chicken and quinoa soup

**Prep time:** 10 minutes
1. Heat 1 tsp olive oil in a saucepan.
2. Add 2 cups low-sodium chicken or vegetable stock.
3. Bring to simmer, add 1 cupped hand quinoa.
4. Add 1 fist of roasted vegetables (chopped smaller).
5. Add 1 palm portion of shredded chicken.
6. Simmer for 5 minutes until heated through.
7. Stir in large handful of fresh spinach (will wilt).
8. Finish with 1 tbsp olive oil and fresh herbs.

**Why this works:** Hydrating + warming + easily digestible + nutrient-dense

## 5. FOUNDATION FOODS FOR YOUR WEEKLY SHOP

- **Eggs:** The ultimate fast food. Always have a box.
- **Greek yogurt:** Your go-to for a high-protein breakfast or snack.
- **Chicken breasts or turkey mince:** Your versatile weekday dinner heroes.
- **Frozen salmon fillets or tinned tuna:** For a quick hit of protein and healthy omega-3 fats.
- **Cottage cheese:** High protein, versatile.
- **Tofu or tempeh:** Versatile protein that takes on any flavour.
- **Lentils (dried or tinned):** Quick-cooking protein and a fibre powerhouse.
- **Chickpeas (tinned):** Perfect for salads, curries or roasted snacks.
- **Hemp seeds or pumpkin seeds:** Easy protein boost for any meal.
- **Coconut yogurt (unsweetened):** For those avoiding dairy.
- **Plant-based protein powder:** Quick breakfast or snack option.
- **Nuts and nut butters:** Almonds, cashews, natural peanut butter.
- **Beans (black, kidney, cannellini):** Affordable protein and high in fibre.
- **A big bag of spinach or rocket:** You can wilt this into anything or use it as a base for a salad in seconds.
- **A head of broccoli:** Versatile, nutrient-dense and brilliant roasted.
- **A bag of frozen mixed peppers:** Already chopped. A lifesaver for stir-fries and omelettes.
- **A bottle of extra-virgin olive oil:** For dressings and drizzling.
- **Avocados:** The king of healthy fats.
- **A bag of almonds or walnuts:** For snacking and sprinkling.
- **A pouch of pre-cooked quinoa or brown rice:** An absolute game-changer for a quick and easy lunch.
- **All sweet potatoes:** More nutrient-dense and gentler on your blood sugar than white ones

- **A bag of frozen berries:** Perfect for adding to yogurt bowls or protein shakes without a huge sugar hit.
- **A bunch of bananas or a bag of apples:** Your easy, portable carb source.

## 6. 10-MINUTE SUPERMARKET SWEEP

**Ready-to-eat protein:** Pre-cooked turkey, ham, chicken strips, salmon; smoked fish; cottage cheese/Greek yogurt; or tinned beans/lentils for plant-based eaters.

**Ready-to-eat veg:**
- Pre-washed mixed salad leaves.
- Pre-chopped 'snacking' veg.

**Ready-to-eat carbs:**
- Pouch of pre-cooked quinoa, lentils or mixed grains.
- Tin of chickpeas.

**Flavouring:** A tub of hummus or a bottle of good-quality vinaigrette.

# ACKNOWLEDGEMENTS

To my mum and brother – thank you for giving me every tool, every push, every reality check and every bit of support I needed to grow. You've helped me build every stage of career, more than you'll ever realise. This book simply wouldn't exist without either of you.

To the team at HarperCollins and my brilliant literary agent – thank you for trusting me, championing my vision and helping me bring this book to life.

To my clients, past, present and future – thank you for your honesty, your vulnerability and your trust. Walking beside you through some of your hardest chapters has changed my life just as much as I hope I've changed yours.

And to you, the reader – if you've tried everything, started over a hundred times or blamed yourself for a body that wouldn't cooperate ... this book is for you. I hope these pages are the moment you finally feel understood.

# NOTES

1   Tosi, Flavia, Bonora, Enzo, and Moghetti, Paolo, 'Insulin resistance in a large cohort of women with polycystic ovary syndrome: A comparison between euglycaemic-hyperinsulinaemic clamp and surrogate indexes'. *Human Reproduction*, December 2017, 32(12):2515–21. https://academic.oup.com/humrep/article/32/12/2515/4523637?utm_source=chatgpt.com&login=false.

2   Saeko, Imai, Kajiyama, Shizuo, Kitta, Kaoru, et al., 'Eating vegetables first regardless of eating speed has a significant reducing effect on postprandial blood glucose and insulin in young healthy women: randomized controlled cross-over study'. 2023, *Nutrients*, 15( 5):1174. https://www.mdpi.com/2072-6643/15/5/1174.

3   Schmid S.M., Hallschmid M., Jauch-Chara K., Born J., and Schultes B., 'A single night of sleep deprivation increases ghrelin levels and feelings of hunger in normal-weight healthy men'. *Journal of Sleep Research*, September 2008, 17(3):331–34. https://pubmed.ncbi.nlm.nih.gov/18564298.

4   Wegner D.M., 'Ironic processes of mental control', *Psychology Review*, January 1994, 101(1):34–52. https://pubmed.ncbi.nlm.nih.gov/8121959.